THE EFFECTS OF PROSTATE CANCER AND ITS PREVENTION

By

Matthias Ziegler

DISCLAIMER

TABLE OF CONTENTS

CHAPTER TWO: CAUSES OF PROSTATE CANCER

Age as a risk factor for prostate cancer

Family history and genetics as a risk factor for prostate cancer

The role of hormones, specifically testosterone, in the development of prostate cancer

Lifestyle factors such as diet, exercise, and smoking in relation to prostate cancer risk

Environmental factors and occupational exposures as potential causes of prostate cancer

Inflammation and its association with prostate cancer development

The link between obesity and increased risk of prostate cancer

PROLOGUE

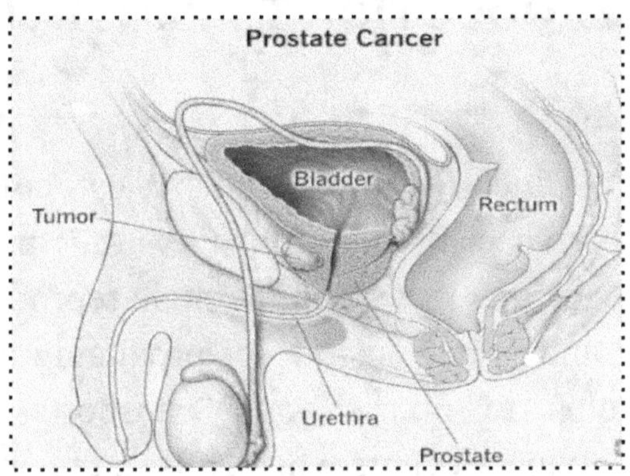

Prostate cancer is a serious health concern for men of all ages. It is the second most common type of cancer in men, and is the leading cause of cancer-related deaths in men. While prostate cancer can be treated successfully if caught early, it can have serious effects if left untreated. In this article, we will discuss the potential effects of prostate cancer and the importance of early detection and treatment. We will also discuss the various treatment options available for prostate cancer and how they can help improve the quality of life for those affected by the disease.

CHAPTER ONE

INTRODUCTION TO PROSTATE CANCER

Prostate cancer is one of the most common forms of cancer in men. It begins in the prostate gland, which is located in the male reproductive system and is responsible for producing a fluid that helps to nourish and transport sperm. Prostate cancer occurs when cells in the prostate gland become abnormal and begin to grow uncontrollably. This abnormal growth can cause the prostate to become enlarged, which can lead to a variety of symptoms, such as difficulty urinating, a decrease in urinary flow, a feeling of incomplete bladder emptying, and blood in the urine.

The exact cause of prostate cancer is unknown, but it is believed to be the result of a combination of factors, including age, race, family history, and diet. Prostate cancer is more common in men over the age of 50 and African-American men, and those with a family history of prostate cancer are at an increased risk. Diet is also thought to play a role in the development of prostate cancer, with diets high in red meat, processed meats, and dairy products being associated with an increased risk.

Prostate cancer can be diagnosed through a variety of tests, including a digital rectal exam, a prostate-specific antigen (PSA) test, a prostate biopsy, and imaging tests such as an MRI or CT scan. Treatment options vary depending on the stage of the cancer, and can include surgery, radiation therapy, hormone therapy, and chemotherapy. If the cancer is in its early stages, it may be possible to treat the cancer with a combination of treatments, such as surgery and radiation therapy.

Prostate cancer is a serious medical condition, and it is important for men to be aware of the risks factors and symptoms associated with the disease, as well as to be proactive in seeking medical care if they are experiencing any changes in their urinary symptoms. Early diagnosis and treatment of prostate cancer can improve outcomes and quality of life.

What is Prostate Cancer and How Does it Affect Men?

Prostate cancer is a malignant tumor that develops in the prostate, a small gland located in the male reproductive system. The prostate is located just in front of the rectum, below the urinary bladder and in front of the rectum. The prostate produces seminal fluid, which helps to nourish and transport sperm.

There are several types of prostate cancer, but the most common type is adenocarcinoma, which starts in the cells of the prostate gland. Other types of prostate cancer include transitional cell carcinoma, small cell carcinoma and sarcomas.

Prostate cancer is a slow-growing cancer, and in many cases, it causes no symptoms at all. If it is detected early, it can be treated and cured. However, if it is left untreated, it can spread to other parts of the body, such as the bones and lymph nodes, leading to serious complications.

The risk factors for prostate cancer include age, family history, race and lifestyle. The risk increases with age, and men aged 65 and older are most likely to develop prostate cancer. Men with a family history of prostate cancer are also at higher risk. African American men are also at higher risk for prostate cancer than other races. Additionally, lifestyle choices, such as a diet high in fat and red meat, can increase the risk of developing prostate cancer.

Prostate cancer can be detected through a physical exam or through a blood test. In a physical exam, the doctor will examine the prostate gland for any abnormalities. In a blood test, the doctor will look for a protein called prostate-specific antigen (PSA) in the blood. High levels of PSA can indicate the presence of prostate cancer.

If prostate cancer is detected, the doctor will recommend a course of treatment. Treatment options include surgery, radiation therapy, hormone therapy, chemotherapy, and immunotherapy. Surgery is the most common treatment option and involves removing the prostate gland and any nearby tissue. Radiation therapy involves using high-energy X-rays to kill cancer cells. Hormone therapy is used to reduce the levels of testosterone in the body, as testosterone can feed prostate cancer cells. Chemotherapy and immunotherapy are used to destroy cancer cells.

The side effects of prostate cancer treatment vary depending on the type of treatment chosen. Surgery can cause urinary incontinence and impotence. Radiation therapy can cause fatigue, diarrhea, and rectal irritation. Hormone therapy can cause hot flashes, decreased sex drive, and breast tenderness. Chemotherapy and immunotherapy can cause nausea and vomiting, hair loss, and fatigue.

Prostate cancer is a serious condition that can have a significant impact on a man's life. Early detection and treatment is essential for a successful outcome. Men should be aware of the risk factors and talk to their doctor about any concerns they have. With the right treatment, prostate cancer can be cured.

The Risk Factors of Prostate Cancer

The risk factors associated with prostate cancer can vary from person to person, and some may not even experience any symptoms until the disease has advanced. Understanding these risk factors is important in identifying those who are at higher risk for prostate cancer, and for early detection and treatment of the disease.

Age is the most significant risk factor for prostate cancer. The risk of developing prostate cancer increases significantly after the age of 50, with most cases occurring in men over the age of 65. This is due to the fact that the prostate gland continues to grow and change throughout a man's life, increasing the likelihood of developing cancerous cells over time.

Family history is also a significant risk factor for prostate cancer. Men with a family history of prostate cancer are two to three times more likely to develop the disease than those without a family history. This risk increases if a man's father or brother has had prostate cancer, particularly if they were diagnosed at a young age. This suggests that there may be a genetic component to the disease.

Ethnicity is another factor that can affect the risk of developing prostate cancer. African-American men are more likely to develop prostate cancer than men of other races, and are also more likely to develop more aggressive forms of the disease. The reasons for this are not yet fully understood, but it may be due to differences in hormone levels or genetic factors.

Diet may also play a role in the development of prostate cancer. A diet high in red meat and dairy products, particularly those that are high in saturated fats, has been linked to an increased risk of prostate cancer. On the other hand, a diet high in fruits, vegetables, and whole grains may help to lower the risk of developing the disease.

Obesity is also a risk factor for prostate cancer. Men who are overweight or obese are more likely to develop the disease than those who are at a healthy weight. This may be due to the fact that obesity can lead to changes in hormone levels, inflammation, and insulin resistance, all of which can contribute to the development of cancer.

Other factors that may increase the risk of prostate cancer include exposure to certain chemicals or toxins, a history of sexually transmitted infections, and a history of other cancers. However, the evidence for these risk factors is not yet conclusive, and more research is needed to fully understand their role in the development of prostate cancer.

In summary, the risk factors for prostate cancer are multifactorial and can vary from person to person. Age, family history, ethnicity, diet, and obesity are among the most significant risk factors for the disease. By understanding these risk factors, men can make lifestyle changes and undergo regular screenings to help prevent the development of prostate cancer or detect it at an early stage.

The Impact of Prostate Cancer on Quality of Life

Prostate cancer is a serious health condition that affects the prostate gland, a walnut-sized organ located below the bladder and in front of the rectum. The impact of prostate cancer on quality of life can be significant, as it may cause a variety of physical, emotional, and social challenges.

Physical Effects:

The physical effects of prostate cancer may include urinary problems such as urinary incontinence, urinary urgency or frequency, difficulty starting or stopping urine flow, and painful urination. Other physical effects may include sexual dysfunction, such as erectile dysfunction, decreased libido, and orgasmic dysfunction. In some cases, prostate cancer may also cause bowel problems, such as diarrhea or constipation.

Emotional Effects:

Prostate cancer can have a significant impact on a person's emotional well-being. The diagnosis of cancer can be a shock and can cause a range of emotional reactions, including anxiety, depression, and fear. These emotions can persist even after treatment has ended, and may affect a person's ability to cope with the illness and its aftermath. Additionally, prostate cancer can cause feelings of shame, embarrassment, and emasculation due to the impact on sexual function.

Social Effects:

Prostate cancer can also have social effects. A person with prostate cancer may need to take time off work for treatment, which can lead to financial strain and difficulties with coworkers or employers. Social isolation can also occur due to the physical and emotional effects of the disease, which can impact personal relationships and social activities.

Coping Strategies:

There are various strategies that can help people with prostate cancer cope with the impact on their quality of life. Seeking support from family, friends, and healthcare professionals can be helpful. Support groups can also provide a safe and supportive environment to share experiences and feelings with others who have prostate cancer. Maintaining a healthy lifestyle, such as regular exercise and a healthy diet, can also help manage some of the physical effects of the disease.

In summary, prostate cancer can have a significant impact on quality of life due to its physical, emotional, and social effects. However, with the help of coping strategies and support, people with prostate cancer can manage the impact of the disease and maintain a good quality of life. It's important to discuss any concerns or challenges with a healthcare professional to receive appropriate treatment and support.

CHAPTER TWO

CAUSES OF PROSTATE CANCER

Prostate cancer occurs when cells in the prostate gland, which is a small gland located in the male reproductive system, grow and divide uncontrollably. The exact cause of prostate cancer is unknown, but it is believed to be the result of a combination of genetic and environmental factors.

Several risk factors have been associated with an increased risk of developing prostate cancer, including age, family history of the disease, ethnicity, and lifestyle factors such as diet and physical activity.

Some studies suggest that changes in certain genes may play a role in the development of prostate cancer. For example, mutations in the BRCA1 and BRCA2 genes, which are known to increase the risk of breast and ovarian cancers in women, may also increase the risk of prostate cancer in men.

Environmental factors, such as exposure to certain chemicals, may also play a role in the development of prostate cancer. However, the evidence linking environmental factors to prostate cancer is not yet conclusive, and more research is needed to fully understand the relationship between the two.

Overall, the exact cause of prostate cancer is not fully understood, but a combination of genetic and environmental factors is believed to play a role in its development.

Age as a risk factor for prostate cancer

Age is a significant risk factor for prostate cancer. The chances of developing prostate cancer increase as a man gets older. According to the American Cancer Society, more than 60% of prostate cancer cases are diagnosed in men aged 65 or older.

In fact, the incidence of prostate cancer is relatively low in men under 50 years old, but it increases sharply after age 50. The risk of developing prostate cancer doubles approximately every 10 years after age 50.

It is not entirely clear why age is such a significant risk factor for prostate cancer, but it is believed that changes in the prostate gland over time may play a role. Additionally, as men age, they may be exposed to more risk factors, such as lifestyle habits, environmental factors, and genetics, that increase their risk of developing prostate cancer.

While age is a significant risk factor, it's important to note that not all older men develop prostate cancer. Regular screening and early detection can help identify prostate cancer in its early stages when treatment is most effective.

Family history and genetics as a risk factor for prostate cancer

Family history and genetics play a significant role in the risk of developing prostate cancer. Having a close relative, such as a father or brother, with prostate cancer can increase your risk of developing the disease. Here are some key points about family history and genetics as risk factors for prostate cancer:

Family History:

Having a first-degree relative (father or brother) with prostate cancer can roughly double your risk of developing the disease compared to individuals with no family history. The risk further increases if multiple relatives are affected or if the affected relative was diagnosed at a young age.

Genetic Mutations:

Certain inherited genetic mutations are associated with an increased risk of prostate cancer. The most well-known mutations linked to prostate cancer are mutations in the BRCA1 and BRCA2 genes, which are commonly associated with breast and ovarian cancers in women. Men with BRCA1 or BRCA2 mutations have a higher risk of developing prostate cancer.

Hereditary Prostate Cancer:

In rare cases, prostate cancer can be inherited in families due to specific gene mutations. These mutations include HOXB13, BRCA1, BRCA2,

ATM, CHEK2, and others. Men with these genetic mutations have an increased risk of developing prostate cancer at an earlier age.

Ethnicity:

Prostate cancer rates vary among different ethnic groups. African-American men have the highest incidence of prostate cancer worldwide, and they are more likely to develop an aggressive form of the disease. Studies suggest that genetic factors may contribute to this higher risk, but the exact genes involved are not yet fully understood.

Shared Lifestyle and Environmental Factors:

In addition to genetic factors, families may share lifestyle and environmental factors that could contribute to prostate cancer risk. These factors can include dietary patterns, exposure to certain chemicals, and similar living environments.

It is important to note that having a family history of prostate cancer or certain genetic mutations does not mean that an individual will definitely develop the disease. It simply indicates an increased risk compared to the general population. Regular screening and early detection are crucial for individuals at higher risk, allowing for timely diagnosis and appropriate treatment, if necessary. If you have concerns about your family history and its potential impact on your risk of prostate cancer, it is advisable to consult with a healthcare professional or genetic counselor who can provide personalized guidance based on your specific situation.

The role of hormones, specifically testosterone, in the development of prostate cancer

Testosterone is a male sex hormone that plays an important role in the development and maintenance of male reproductive tissues, including the prostate gland. However, there is evidence to suggest that high levels of testosterone may also contribute to the development of prostate cancer.

Prostate cancer is the most common cancer among men, and it is estimated that about one in eight men will develop the disease at some point in their lives. Although the exact causes of prostate cancer are not fully understood, it is known that the growth and survival of prostate cancer cells are dependent on the male hormone testosterone.

Testosterone is produced by the testes and adrenal glands, and it is converted to dihydrotestosterone (DHT) in the prostate gland. DHT is a more potent form of testosterone that is responsible for promoting the growth and function of prostate cells.

The role of testosterone in the development of prostate cancer is complex and not fully understood. It is thought that high levels of testosterone may contribute to the development of prostate cancer by stimulating the growth and division of cancerous cells in the prostate gland.

However, there is also evidence to suggest that low levels of testosterone may also increase the risk of developing prostate cancer. This may be because testosterone plays a protective role in the prostate gland, and low levels of the hormone may lead to an increased risk of cellular damage and mutations that can lead to cancer.

In addition to testosterone, other hormones such as estrogen and progesterone may also play a role in the development of prostate cancer. These hormones are typically associated with female reproductive function, but they are also present in men at lower levels.

Overall, the role of hormones in the development of prostate cancer is complex and multifactorial. While testosterone is known to play an important role in the growth and function of the prostate gland, the relationship between testosterone and prostate cancer is not fully understood and requires further study.

Lifestyle factors such as diet, exercise, and smoking in relation to prostate cancer risk

Lifestyle factors such as diet, exercise, and smoking can indeed influence the risk of developing prostate cancer. While the exact causes of prostate cancer are still not fully understood, research suggests that adopting a healthy lifestyle can help reduce the risk of developing this disease. Here's a breakdown of how these factors relate to prostate cancer risk:

Diet:

A healthy diet can play a significant role in reducing prostate cancer risk. Some dietary recommendations to consider include:

- **Fruits and vegetables:** Consuming a variety of fruits and vegetables, particularly those rich in antioxidants, is beneficial. These include berries, leafy greens, tomatoes, and cruciferous vegetables like broccoli and cauliflower.

- **Healthy fats:** Opt for healthy fats such as those found in fish (especially fatty fish like salmon), nuts, seeds, and olive oil. These fats contain omega-3 fatty acids, which have been associated with a lower risk of prostate cancer.

- **Limit red meat and processed foods:** High intake of red and processed meats has been linked to an increased risk of prostate cancer. It's advisable to moderate the consumption of these foods.

- **Soy products:** Some studies suggest that soy products like tofu, tempeh, and soy milk may have a protective effect against prostate cancer. However, more research is needed to establish a conclusive link.

Exercise:

Regular physical activity is beneficial for overall health and may also reduce the risk of prostate cancer. Engaging in moderate to vigorous exercise, such as brisk walking, jogging, swimming, or cycling, for at least 150 minutes per week is generally recommended.

Smoking:

Smoking is a well-known risk factor for various types of cancer, including prostate cancer. Research suggests that smokers may have a higher risk of developing aggressive prostate cancer compared to non-smokers. Quitting smoking or avoiding it altogether can significantly lower the risk.

It's worth noting that while lifestyle modifications can contribute to reducing the risk of prostate cancer, they do not guarantee prevention. Other factors such as genetics, age, and family history also play a role. Regular check-ups, including prostate-specific antigen (PSA) testing and discussions with a healthcare professional, are crucial for early detection and appropriate management of prostate cancer.

Environmental factors and occupational exposures as potential causes of prostate cancer

Prostate cancer is a complex disease, and its exact causes are not fully understood. While the primary risk factors for prostate cancer include age, family history, and genetics, there is ongoing research investigating the role of environmental factors and occupational exposures in its development. Here are some potential factors that have been studied:

Environmental Chemicals:

Certain environmental chemicals, such as pesticides, heavy metals, and organic solvents, have been investigated for their potential link to prostate cancer. Prolonged exposure to these substances, especially in occupational settings, may increase the risk. However, the evidence is still limited, and further research is needed to establish a clear association.

Air Pollution:

Several studies have examined the relationship between air pollution and prostate cancer. Long-term exposure to air pollutants, including particulate matter and certain gases, has been associated with a higher risk of prostate cancer. However, the evidence is not yet conclusive, and more research is required to better understand this relationship.

Diet and Lifestyle:

While not strictly environmental factors, diet and lifestyle choices can impact the risk of prostate cancer. High consumption of red and processed meats, low intake of fruits and vegetables, obesity, and sedentary behavior have been linked to an increased risk. Conversely, a healthy diet rich in plant-based foods, regular physical activity, and maintaining a healthy weight may reduce the risk of developing prostate cancer.

Occupational Exposures:

Some occupational exposures have been suggested to contribute to prostate cancer risk. For instance, firefighters, farmers, and individuals working in the rubber, cadmium, or welding industries may face higher risks due to specific exposures encountered in their work environments. However, further studies are necessary to establish a definitive causal relationship.

Radiation Exposure:

Prolonged or repeated exposure to ionizing radiation, such as medical radiation treatments or occupational radiation exposure, may increase the risk of prostate cancer. However, the risk associated with medical radiation is generally low, and the benefits of necessary medical procedures often outweigh the potential risks.

It is important to note that while these factors have been investigated, the evidence is not yet conclusive, and more research is needed to establish their precise role in prostate cancer development. Additionally, prostate cancer is a complex disease influenced by multiple factors, including genetic and hormonal influences. Regular screenings and early detection remain crucial in managing and treating prostate cancer.

Inflammation and its association with prostate cancer development

Inflammation is a complex biological response triggered by the immune system in response to harmful stimuli such as pathogens, tissue damage, or irritants. While inflammation is a natural defense mechanism, chronic or prolonged inflammation can have detrimental effects on the body and has been associated with the development and progression of various diseases, including cancer.

Prostate cancer is the most common non-skin cancer in men and is characterized by the abnormal growth of cells in the prostate gland. The exact causes of prostate cancer are not fully understood, but research has suggested that chronic inflammation may play a role in its development. Here are a few key points about the association between inflammation and prostate cancer:

Inflammatory Conditions:

Certain inflammatory conditions, such as chronic prostatitis (inflammation of the prostate) and benign prostatic hyperplasia (BPH), have been linked to an increased risk of developing prostate cancer. However, it's important to note that not all cases of inflammation or these conditions lead to prostate cancer.

Immune Response:

Inflammation involves the activation of immune cells, such as macrophages and T cells, which release various signaling molecules (cytokines, chemokines) and reactive oxygen species.

These factors can promote DNA damage, cell proliferation, and angiogenesis (formation of new blood vessels), which are all processes that can contribute to cancer development.

Chronic Inflammation and DNA Damage:

Prolonged inflammation can lead to the production of reactive oxygen species and reactive nitrogen species, which can cause DNA damage. DNA damage, if not properly repaired, can result in genetic mutations that may contribute to the development of cancer, including prostate cancer.

Inflammatory Mediators:

Inflammatory mediators, such as interleukins (IL-1, IL-6), tumor necrosis factor-alpha (TNF-α), and cyclooxygenase-2 (COX-2), have been found to be elevated in both prostate tissue and blood of individuals with prostate cancer. These mediators can promote cell growth, survival, and angiogenesis, and they may contribute to the development and progression of prostate cancer.

Inflammatory Markers:

Elevated levels of certain inflammatory markers, such as C-reactive protein (CRP) and prostaglandin E2 (PGE2), have been associated with an increased risk of prostate cancer and worse clinical outcomes. These markers can serve as indicators of the presence and severity of inflammation in the body.

While the association between inflammation and prostate cancer is evident, it is essential to understand that inflammation alone does not cause cancer. Other factors, including genetic predisposition, hormonal imbalances, and lifestyle factors, also play crucial roles in prostate cancer development. Nonetheless, targeting inflammation and its mediators may hold promise for the prevention and treatment of prostate cancer in the future. It's always important to consult with a healthcare professional for personalized advice and screenings related to prostate health and cancer.

The link between obesity and increased risk of prostate cancer

There is evidence to suggest that obesity is associated with an increased risk of prostate cancer. Several studies have found a positive correlation between obesity and the development, progression, and aggressiveness of prostate cancer. Here are some key points regarding the link between obesity and prostate cancer risk:

Incidence:

Obese individuals have a higher risk of developing prostate cancer compared to those with a healthy weight. The risk appears to be particularly elevated for advanced or aggressive forms of the disease.

Progression and Aggressiveness:

Obesity may contribute to the progression and aggressiveness of prostate cancer. Obese men are more likely to have larger tumors, higher-grade tumors, and a greater likelihood of the cancer spreading beyond the prostate gland.

Hormonal Factors:

Obesity is associated with alterations in hormone levels, including increased levels of insulin and estrogen, and decreased levels of testosterone. These hormonal changes may promote the growth of prostate cancer cells.

Inflammation:

Obesity is characterized by a chronic state of inflammation. Inflammation has been linked to various cancers, including prostate cancer. It is believed that the inflammatory environment in obese individuals may contribute to the development and progression of prostate cancer.

Treatment Challenges:

Obesity can pose challenges in the treatment of prostate cancer. It may affect the accuracy of diagnostic tests, such as prostate-specific antigen (PSA) tests, due to higher blood volumes and increased PSA levels associated with obesity. Additionally, obese individuals may face difficulties in surgery and radiation treatment, and they may experience higher rates of treatment-related complications.

While the exact mechanisms underlying the link between obesity and prostate cancer are not fully understood, it is generally recommended for individuals to maintain a healthy weight through a balanced diet and regular exercise. This not only helps in reducing the risk of prostate cancer but also offers numerous other health benefits. If you have concerns about your prostate health, it is always advisable to consult with a healthcare professional for personalized advice and appropriate screenings.

The role of chronic diseases such as diabetes in the development of prostate cancer

Chronic diseases, including diabetes, can potentially influence the development and progression of prostate cancer, although the exact relationship between the two is not yet fully understood. Several studies have investigated the potential link between diabetes and prostate cancer, and while some have suggested an association, others have not found a clear relationship. Here are some key points to consider:

Insulin Resistance:

Diabetes is characterized by insulin resistance, where the body's cells become less responsive to the effects of insulin. Insulin is a hormone that regulates blood sugar levels, but it also has growth-promoting properties. Some research suggests that high insulin levels or insulin resistance may contribute to the development of certain cancers, including prostate cancer.

Inflammation:

Chronic inflammation is another common feature of both diabetes and cancer. Inflammation can create an environment that promotes the growth and spread of cancer cells. It is believed that the persistent inflammation associated with diabetes might contribute to the development of prostate cancer.

Shared Risk Factors:

Diabetes and prostate cancer share some common risk factors, such as age, obesity, and sedentary lifestyle. These factors may independently increase the risk of both conditions. It is important to note that these risk factors are associated with an increased likelihood of developing many chronic diseases, including various types of cancer.

Detection Bias:

Some studies suggest that the observed association between diabetes and prostate cancer might be influenced by detection bias. Diabetic individuals may undergo more regular medical check-ups, including prostate-specific antigen (PSA) testing, which could lead to an increased likelihood of diagnosing prostate cancer.

Treatment Challenges:

If a person with diabetes is diagnosed with prostate cancer, managing both conditions simultaneously can present challenges. The treatment of prostate cancer, such as certain hormonal therapies, may affect glucose metabolism and insulin sensitivity, potentially complicating diabetes management.

It's important to note that while some studies have found a link between diabetes and prostate cancer, others have not established a clear association. The relationship between chronic diseases like diabetes and prostate cancer is complex and influenced by various factors. More research is needed to fully understand the underlying mechanisms and determine the extent of the association between these conditions. If you have specific concerns or questions, it's best to consult with a healthcare professional who can provide personalized guidance based on your individual situation.

Prostate cancer screening and its impact on early detection and prevention

Prostate cancer screening plays a crucial role in the early detection and prevention of prostate cancer. Early detection is essential because it increases the chances of successful treatment and improves overall prognosis. Let's explore the different screening methods and their impact:

Digital Rectal Examination (DRE):

During a DRE, a healthcare provider manually examines the prostate gland by inserting a gloved, lubricated finger into the rectum. Although it is a relatively simple procedure, it allows the doctor to feel for any abnormalities, such as lumps or hard areas, which might indicate the presence of prostate cancer. DRE is often combined with other screening methods for better accuracy.

Prostate-Specific Antigen (PSA) Test:

The PSA test measures the levels of a protein called prostate-specific antigen in the blood. Elevated PSA levels can be an indication of prostate cancer, but they can also be caused by non-cancerous conditions like prostatitis or benign prostatic hyperplasia (BPH). While the PSA test is not perfect and can sometimes yield false-positive results, it remains a valuable tool for detecting prostate cancer early.

The impact of prostate cancer screening on early detection and prevention can be seen in the following ways:

- **Early Detection:**
  Regular screening enables the detection of prostate cancer at an early stage, often before any noticeable symptoms develop. This allows for timely intervention and treatment, which can significantly improve outcomes. When diagnosed early, prostate cancer has a higher chance of being localized and potentially curable.

- **Increased Survival Rates:**
  Early detection through screening has been associated with increased survival rates for prostate cancer. Treatment options such as surgery, radiation therapy, hormone therapy, and chemotherapy are more effective when the cancer is localized and has not spread beyond the prostate gland.

- **Personalized Treatment Approach:** Early detection facilitates a personalized approach to treatment. By identifying the cancer at an early stage, healthcare professionals can determine the most suitable treatment options for each patient based on their specific condition and overall health. This may help avoid unnecessary overtreatment or choose the best course of action.

- **Monitoring High-Risk Individuals:** Prostate cancer screening is particularly crucial for individuals at higher risk, such as those with a family history of the disease or African American men who have a higher incidence rate. Regular screening allows close monitoring of these individuals and enables the detection of prostate cancer at an earlier stage, when it is most treatable.

It is important to note that while prostate cancer screening has benefits, it also has limitations. False-positive results can lead to unnecessary biopsies and potential complications. Additionally, the decision to undergo prostate cancer screening should be based on an individual's risk factors, age, and preferences. It is recommended to have a discussion with a healthcare professional to understand the benefits and potential drawbacks of screening in each specific case.

The potential impact of certain medications and supplements on prostate cancer risk.

The impact of medications and supplements on prostate cancer risk is a complex topic, and research in this area is ongoing. While some substances have shown potential effects on prostate cancer risk, it is important to note that the available evidence is often preliminary, and more research is needed to establish clear conclusions. Here are some medications and supplements that have been investigated:

- **5-alpha-reductase inhibitors (Finasteride, Dutasteride):** These medications are commonly used to treat benign prostatic hyperplasia (BPH) and hair loss. Studies have shown that these drugs may reduce the risk of developing low-grade prostate cancer. However, they may also increase the risk of developing higher-grade and more aggressive prostate cancer. As a result, the use of these medications for prostate cancer prevention is still controversial.

- **Nonsteroidal anti-inflammatory drugs (NSAIDs):**
  Some research suggests that NSAIDs, such as aspirin, may have a protective effect against prostate cancer. Regular use of NSAIDs has been associated with a reduced risk of developing aggressive prostate cancer. However, more studies are needed to confirm these findings and determine the optimal dosage and duration of use.

- **Vitamin E:**
  Vitamin E has been studied extensively for its potential role in preventing prostate cancer. However, large clinical trials such as the SELECT trial found that vitamin E supplementation (in the form of alpha-tocopherol) did not reduce the risk of prostate cancer and, in some

cases, may have slightly increased the risk.

- **Selenium:**

Selenium is a trace mineral that has been investigated for its potential protective effects against prostate cancer. Results from studies have been mixed, with some suggesting a possible reduction in risk, particularly in individuals with low selenium levels. However, other studies have not shown a significant effect.

- **Lycopene:**

Lycopene is a carotenoid found in tomatoes and other fruits. It has been studied for its potential role in reducing prostate cancer risk. Some evidence suggests that higher intake of lycopene-rich foods or supplements may be associated with a lower risk of prostate cancer, particularly aggressive forms. However, more research is needed to establish a definitive link.

It is important to note that these substances should not be used as a replacement for standard medical care. If you have concerns about your prostate health or are at an increased risk of prostate cancer, it is recommended to consult with a healthcare professional who can provide personalized advice based on your specific circumstances.

CHAPTER THREE

SYMPTOMS OF PROSTATE CANCER

Prostate cancer is a type of cancer that occurs in the prostate gland, which is a small walnut-shaped gland in men that produces seminal fluid. Prostate cancer often develops slowly and may not cause noticeable symptoms in the early stages. However, as the cancer progresses, it can cause various symptoms. Here are some common symptoms associated with prostate cancer:

- ☐ Urinary problems
- ☐ Erectile dysfunction
- ☐ Blood in semen
- ☐ Pain and discomfort
- ☐ Weight loss and fatigue

Early-stage Symptoms Of Prostate Cancer

Prostate cancer is a common form of cancer that affects the prostate gland, which is a small walnut-shaped gland located below the bladder in men. In its early stages, prostate cancer may not cause noticeable symptoms. However, there are some initial signs and symptoms that may indicate the presence of prostate cancer. These symptoms include frequent urination, difficulty starting or stopping urination, weak urine flow, and blood in the urine or semen.

Frequent urination is a symptom that may occur in the early stages of prostate cancer. Men may find themselves needing to urinate more often than usual, particularly during the night. This can be attributed to the enlargement of the prostate gland, which can put pressure on the urethra, the tube that carries urine from the bladder out of the body. As a result, the bladder may not empty completely, leading to more frequent urges to urinate.

Difficulty starting or stopping urination is another common symptom of prostate cancer. Men with prostate cancer may experience a delay or hesitation when trying to initiate urination. Likewise, they may find it challenging to completely empty their bladder or may have a weak urine stream. These difficulties arise due to the obstruction caused by an enlarged prostate, which can impede the normal flow of urine.

A weak urine flow can also be indicative of prostate cancer. Instead of a strong, forceful stream, men with prostate cancer may notice a reduced flow or a stream that appears weaker than usual. This weakened urine flow is again a consequence of the enlarged prostate gland, which can constrict the urethra and impede the normal passage of urine.

In some cases, blood in the urine or semen may be an early sign of prostate cancer. This symptom, known as hematuria or hematospermia respectively, can be alarming and should be evaluated by a healthcare professional. While blood in the urine or semen can occur due to various reasons other than prostate cancer, it is still important to rule out prostate cancer as a potential cause.

It is worth noting that these early-stage symptoms of prostate cancer are not specific to the disease and can also be caused by other conditions such as benign prostatic hyperplasia (BPH) or urinary tract infections. However, if any of these symptoms persist or worsen over time, it is crucial to consult a healthcare provider for further evaluation and appropriate testing.

Prostate cancer is often asymptomatic in its early stages, making regular screenings and check-ups important, especially for men above the age of 50 or those with a family history of the disease. Screening methods such as the prostate-specific antigen (PSA) blood test and digital rectal examination (DRE) can help detect prostate cancer at an early stage, even before symptoms manifest.

In conclusion, the early-stage symptoms of prostate cancer may include frequent urination, difficulty starting or stopping urination, weak urine flow, and blood in the urine or semen. However, it is essential to note that these symptoms can also be attributed to other conditions, and only a healthcare professional can provide an accurate diagnosis through appropriate evaluation and testing. Regular screenings and check-ups are vital for the early detection and effective management of prostate cancer.

Advanced-stage symptoms of prostate cancer

Prostate cancer is a malignant condition that primarily affects the prostate gland, a small walnut-shaped organ located below the bladder in men. As the disease progresses to advanced stages, it can manifest various severe symptoms that significantly impact a person's health and well-being. In this essay, I will delve into the advanced-stage symptoms of prostate cancer, highlighting bone pain, weight loss, fatigue, urinary incontinence, erectile dysfunction, and bowel obstruction.

Bone pain is a common symptom experienced by individuals with advanced-stage prostate cancer. The cancer cells can metastasize, or spread, to the bones, leading to bone metastases. The bones most commonly affected include the spine, pelvis, hips, and long bones of the legs. Metastatic bone lesions can cause severe pain, often described as aching, throbbing, or sharp. The pain can become progressively worse and may limit mobility, impacting daily activities and overall quality of life.

Weight loss is another significant symptom associated with advanced-stage prostate cancer. Cancer cells can interfere with the normal metabolic processes of the body, leading to unintentional weight loss. Additionally, the disease may cause a decrease in appetite, making it difficult for patients to consume an adequate amount of calories. Unexplained weight loss is concerning as it can further weaken the body, reduce muscle mass, and contribute to fatigue.

Fatigue is a prevalent symptom in advanced prostate cancer. The cancerous cells, along with the body's immune response, can drain the individual's energy levels, resulting in persistent and overwhelming fatigue. This fatigue is often more severe than regular tiredness and can be debilitating, limiting a person's ability to carry out everyday tasks.

Urinary incontinence is a distressing symptom that may occur as prostate cancer progresses. The growing tumor can press against the urethra, the tube that carries urine from the bladder out of the body, leading to urinary problems. This can result in urinary incontinence, characterized by the inability to control urine flow, leakage, or frequent urination. In some cases, urinary obstruction may occur, causing acute urinary retention, which necessitates immediate medical intervention.

Erectile dysfunction is another challenging symptom experienced by men with advanced-stage prostate cancer. The cancerous growth or its treatment methods, such as surgery, radiation, or hormone therapy, can disrupt the normal blood flow and nerve function required for achieving and maintaining an erection. Erectile dysfunction can significantly impact a man's self-esteem, relationships, and overall quality of life.

Bowel obstruction is a less common but potentially severe symptom of advanced-stage prostate cancer. The tumor can grow and exert pressure on the rectum or colon, leading to a partial or complete blockage. This can result in symptoms such as abdominal pain, bloating, constipation, or the inability to pass stool or gas. Bowel obstruction requires immediate medical attention as it can lead to complications such as bowel perforation or infection.

In conclusion, advanced-stage prostate cancer can give rise to a range of severe symptoms that significantly impact a person's physical and emotional well-being. These symptoms may include bone pain, weight loss, fatigue, urinary incontinence, erectile dysfunction, and bowel obstruction. It is crucial for individuals experiencing these symptoms to seek medical attention promptly to receive appropriate management and support. Additionally, caregivers and healthcare providers play a vital role in providing comprehensive care and addressing the physical and psychological challenges faced by those living with advanced prostate cancer.

Non-specific symptoms of prostate cancer

While prostate cancer often presents with specific symptoms such as urinary difficulties, blood in urine or semen, and erectile dysfunction, there are certain non-specific symptoms that may indicate the presence of the disease. It is crucial to recognize and seek medical attention for these non-specific symptoms, as they could potentially be early signs of prostate cancer or other underlying health conditions. This article aims to shed light on four non-specific symptoms: general discomfort in the pelvic area, lower back pain, unexplained weight loss, and changes in appetite.

General Discomfort in the Pelvic Area:

Men experiencing general discomfort or pain in the pelvic area should be aware that it can be associated with prostate cancer. The prostate gland is located in the pelvic region, and when cancer develops, it can cause inflammation and pressure on surrounding tissues. This may result in a dull ache or discomfort in the pelvic area, which can extend to the lower abdomen, groin, or perineum. While this symptom is not exclusive to prostate cancer and can have other causes, such as inflammation or infection, it is advisable to consult a healthcare professional to determine the underlying cause and rule out prostate cancer.

Lower Back Pain:

Lower back pain is a common complaint among individuals of all ages, but when experienced in conjunction with other symptoms, it may warrant medical attention. Prostate cancer can spread to the bones, including the spine, leading to localized pain or discomfort in the lower back. This pain may worsen over time, become more persistent, or be unrelated to physical exertion or injury. While various factors can contribute to lower back pain, it is essential to consider prostate cancer as a potential cause, especially in men over the age of 50. A thorough evaluation by a healthcare provider can help identify the cause and provide appropriate management.

Unexplained Weight Loss:

Unexplained weight loss refers to a significant decrease in body weight without intentional changes in diet or physical activity. While weight loss can be attributed to a range of factors, including stress or metabolic disorders, it can also be an indicator of an underlying health issue, such as prostate cancer. Cancer cells consume a significant amount of energy, leading to unintended weight loss. When combined with other symptoms or risk factors for prostate cancer, such as age and family history, unexplained weight loss should not be ignored. Consultation with a healthcare professional is essential to identify the cause and initiate appropriate investigations.

Changes in Appetite:

Changes in appetite, such as a sudden loss of interest in food or a persistent decrease in appetite, can be subtle yet significant signs of an underlying health condition. Prostate cancer, like other forms of cancer, can affect the body's metabolism and lead to changes in appetite. These changes may manifest as a lack of interest in meals, early satiety, or a decrease in food consumption resulting in unintended weight loss. Monitoring and reporting changes in appetite to a healthcare provider can help identify potential causes, including prostate cancer, and prompt further evaluation.

In conclusion while general discomfort in the pelvic area, lower back pain, unexplained weight loss, and changes in appetite are non-specific symptoms that may not be directly linked to prostate cancer, they can still warrant medical attention. It is crucial to recognize that these symptoms can result from various underlying causes, including prostate cancer, as well as other health conditions. Consulting a healthcare professional for a comprehensive evaluation is essential to determine the underlying cause and provide appropriate diagnosis and treatment. Timely detection and management of prostate cancer greatly improve the chances of successful outcomes and overall well-being.

Metastatic prostate cancer symptoms

Metastatic prostate cancer occurs when prostate cancer cells spread beyond the prostate gland and invade other parts of the body. As the cancer spreads, it can affect various areas, leading to a range of symptoms. These symptoms can vary depending on the specific organs or areas affected by the cancer. In this essay, we will explore the common symptoms associated with metastatic prostate cancer and discuss their significance.

One of the most common sites of metastasis in prostate cancer is the bones. When cancer cells spread to the bones, they can weaken the bone structure, making them more prone to fractures. Therefore, one of the primary symptoms of metastatic prostate cancer is bone fractures. Patients may experience sudden or unexplained bone pain, particularly in the spine, hips, and pelvis. The pain may worsen with movement and can be severe. Fractures caused by metastatic prostate cancer are often referred to as pathological fractures.

Another significant symptom of metastatic prostate cancer is spinal cord compression. When cancer spreads to the spine, it can put pressure on the spinal cord and nerves, resulting in compression. This can lead to severe back pain, numbness or weakness in the legs, difficulty walking, and problems with bladder or bowel function. Spinal cord compression is a medical emergency requiring immediate attention to prevent permanent damage.

Lymph node enlargement is another common manifestation of metastatic prostate cancer.

Lymph nodes are small, bean-shaped structures that play a crucial role in the immune system. When prostate cancer spreads to the lymph nodes, they can become enlarged and palpable. Enlarged lymph nodes may be felt as lumps under the skin, particularly in the groin, neck, or underarm regions. However, it's important to note that lymph node enlargement can also occur due to other conditions, so further evaluation is necessary to confirm its cause.

Metastatic prostate cancer can also affect specific organs or areas, leading to symptoms related to those particular sites. For example, if the cancer spreads to the liver, it can cause jaundice (yellowing of the skin and eyes), abdominal pain, and weight loss. If the cancer affects the lungs, it may cause coughing, shortness of breath, chest pain, or even coughing up blood. When cancer spreads to the brain, it can cause headaches, seizures, dizziness, or changes in mental function.

Apart from these specific symptoms, metastatic prostate cancer can also cause generalized symptoms that are not necessarily related to a specific site of metastasis. These symptoms may include fatigue, unintentional weight loss, loss of appetite, and generalized pain.

It's important to note that not all individuals with metastatic prostate cancer will experience the same symptoms, and the severity of symptoms can vary widely. Some individuals may have no symptoms at all, especially in the early stages of metastasis. Therefore, regular check-ups and monitoring are crucial for early detection and appropriate management.

In conclusion, metastatic prostate cancer can lead to a variety of symptoms depending on the organs or areas affected by the cancer. Bone fractures, spinal cord compression, lymph node enlargement, and symptoms related to specific organs are commonly observed. These symptoms can significantly impact a patient's quality of life and require prompt medical attention. Early detection and appropriate management are essential for improving outcomes and providing the best possible care for individuals with metastatic prostate cancer.

Rare symptoms and complications of prostate cancer

Prostate cancer is often present with common symptoms such as urinary difficulties, pain, and erectile dysfunction, there are rare symptoms and complications that can arise in some cases. These unusual manifestations can be indicative of advanced disease or a more aggressive form of prostate cancer. Furthermore, potential complications can arise due to the disease itself or its treatment, affecting various aspects of a patient's health and well-being.

Rare symptoms associated with prostate cancer may include anemia, jaundice, neurological symptoms, and paraneoplastic syndromes. Anemia, characterized by a decrease in red blood cells or hemoglobin levels, may occur due to chronic bleeding within the prostate gland or bone marrow infiltration by cancer cells. Symptoms of anemia can manifest as fatigue, weakness, shortness of breath, and pale skin.

Jaundice, a yellowing of the skin and eyes, can be a rare sign of advanced prostate cancer. It may occur when cancer spreads to the liver, causing bile duct obstruction. This obstruction leads to the accumulation of bilirubin, a yellow pigment produced by the liver, resulting in jaundice. In addition to yellowing, other symptoms may include dark urine, pale stools, abdominal pain, and generalized itching.

Neurological symptoms associated with prostate cancer are relatively uncommon but can occur if the cancer spreads to the spine or brain. Compression of the spinal cord or nerves can lead to symptoms such as back pain, weakness or numbness in the limbs, difficulty walking, and loss of bowel or bladder control. In more advanced cases, metastatic lesions in the brain can cause headaches, seizures, cognitive changes, and neurological deficits specific to the affected areas.

Paraneoplastic syndromes are rare manifestations that arise due to substances released by cancer cells or an abnormal immune response triggered by the tumor. Prostate cancer can cause paraneoplastic syndromes such as hypercalcemia, which is characterized by high levels of calcium in the blood. This can lead to symptoms like fatigue, confusion, constipation, nausea, and excessive thirst. Other paraneoplastic syndromes associated with prostate cancer include hypertrophic osteoarthropathy, gynecomastia, and Cushing's syndrome.

Complications of prostate cancer can extend beyond the physical symptoms of the disease itself. Urinary tract infections (UTIs) can occur due to urinary obstruction caused by an enlarged prostate or urinary catheter use. These infections can result in symptoms like painful urination, frequent urge to urinate, lower abdominal pain, and fever. Prompt treatment with antibiotics is crucial to prevent the spread of infection to the kidneys, which can lead to more severe complications.

Prostate cancer can also affect the bladder and kidneys directly. Urinary retention, where the bladder is unable to empty completely, may occur due to obstruction or nerve damage. This can lead to urinary frequency, urgency, nocturia (frequent urination at night), and a weak urine stream. Additionally, kidney problems can arise when cancer spreads to the kidneys or obstructs the urinary tract, potentially causing hydronephrosis (swelling of the kidneys), kidney stones, or kidney failure.

Psychologically, a prostate cancer diagnosis can have a significant impact on a patient's emotional well-being. The news of having cancer and the uncertainties associated with its prognosis and treatment can lead to feelings of anxiety, fear, depression, and stress. Coping with the potential side effects of treatment, changes in body image, sexual dysfunction, and concerns about mortality can further contribute to psychological distress. It is essential for patients to have access to psychological support, counseling, and support groups to address these challenges and maintain overall well-being.

CHAPTER FOUR

DIAGNOSIS AND TESTS FOR PROSTATE CANCER

The diagnosis and testing methods for prostate cancer have undergone significant advancements, leading to improvements in the detection and management of this disease. Here are some key areas where these improvements have occurred:

Early detection:

Early detection is crucial for successful treatment outcomes. Prostate-specific antigen (PSA) blood test is a widely used screening tool for prostate cancer. Recent advancements in PSA testing include refinements in cutoff levels and the development of more sensitive PSA tests, such as the free-to-total PSA ratio. These improvements help in identifying prostate cancer at an earlier stage when it is more likely to be curable.

Imaging techniques:

Various imaging technologies have advanced the diagnosis of prostate cancer. Multiparametric Magnetic Resonance Imaging (mpMRI) is now commonly used to visualize the prostate gland and detect suspicious areas. It provides detailed anatomical information and helps guide targeted biopsies. mpMRI has higher sensitivity and specificity than traditional transrectal ultrasound-guided biopsies, reducing unnecessary biopsies and improving the accuracy of cancer detection.

Biomarkers:

Researchers have identified and validated several biomarkers that can aid in diagnosing prostate cancer. These biomarkers include genetic markers, RNA/DNA signatures, and proteins found in blood, urine, or tissue samples. By analyzing these biomarkers, healthcare professionals can assess the presence, aggressiveness, and progression of prostate cancer. These tests complement traditional diagnostic methods and help in making informed treatment decisions.

Liquid biopsies:

Liquid biopsies involve analyzing circulating tumor cells (CTCs) or tumor-specific DNA fragments found in blood samples. These non-invasive tests can provide information about the genetic characteristics of prostate tumors, monitor treatment response, and detect the development of resistance. Liquid biopsies have the potential to replace or complement traditional tissue biopsies, allowing for more frequent monitoring and personalized treatment approaches.

Genetic testing:

Advances in genetic testing have improved our understanding of the genetic factors involved in prostate cancer development. Testing for specific genetic mutations, such as BRCA1 and BRCA2, can help identify individuals at a higher risk of developing prostate cancer. Additionally, genetic testing can guide treatment decisions, such as the use of targeted therapies or immunotherapies, based on the genetic profile of the tumor.

Artificial intelligence (AI):

AI techniques, such as machine learning and deep learning, are being utilized to analyze large datasets and improve the accuracy of prostate cancer diagnosis. AI algorithms can analyze medical images, pathology slides, and patient data to identify patterns and predict outcomes. These technologies have the potential to assist healthcare professionals in making more accurate diagnoses and personalized treatment recommendations.

Overall, the improvements in diagnosis and testing for prostate cancer have led to more precise and individualized management strategies. Early detection, enhanced imaging techniques, the use of biomarkers and genetic testing, liquid biopsies, and the integration of AI technologies have collectively contributed to better patient outcomes, reduced unnecessary procedures, and improved treatment decision-making in prostate cancer care.

Prostate-Specific Antigen (PSA) Test

The PSA (prostate-specific antigen) test is a common diagnostic tool used to screen for prostate cancer. It measures the amount of PSA protein in a man's blood, which is produced by the prostate gland. PSA levels can be elevated due to various reasons, including prostate cancer, prostatitis (inflammation of the prostate gland), and benign prostatic hyperplasia (enlargement of the prostate gland).

The procedure for the PSA test is simple and involves taking a blood sample from the patient. The sample is then sent to a laboratory where it is analyzed for PSA levels. It is recommended that men over the age of 50 or men with a family history of prostate cancer should undergo the PSA test annually.

The significance of PSA levels lies in the fact that an elevated PSA level may indicate the presence of prostate cancer. However, it is important to note that a high PSA level does not always mean that a person has cancer. In fact, many men with elevated PSA levels do not have prostate cancer.

The interpretation of PSA test results requires careful consideration of a patient's individual situation, including age, family history, and any prior prostate health issues. A normal PSA level is typically considered to be 4 ng/mL or lower. However, it is important to note that there is no specific cutoff for what constitutes a "normal" PSA level. Doctors may consider additional factors such as PSA velocity (how quickly PSA levels rise over time) and PSA density (the PSA level relative to the size of the prostate gland) when interpreting test results.

If a patient's PSA levels are elevated, further testing may be necessary to determine the cause. This may include a digital rectal exam (DRE), imaging tests such as an ultrasound or MRI, or a biopsy of the prostate gland. A biopsy is the only way to definitively diagnose prostate cancer.

In summary, the PSA test is a common diagnostic tool used to screen for prostate cancer. While an elevated PSA level may indicate the presence of prostate cancer, it is important to interpret test results in the context of a patient's individual situation and consider additional testing to confirm a diagnosis.

Digital Rectal Examination (DRE)

A digital rectal examination (DRE) is a procedure used in the diagnosis of prostate cancer. It involves a healthcare professional inserting a gloved, lubricated finger into the rectum to assess the size, shape, and texture of the prostate gland. While a DRE is a useful tool in the diagnosis of prostate cancer, it is not sufficient as a standalone screening method. Here's an overview of the procedure, its purpose, and its limitations:

Procedure:

- **Preparation:**
  The patient is usually asked to lie on their side with their knees drawn up toward their chest or bend over an examination table. The healthcare professional will then put on a lubricated glove and apply lubricant to their finger.

☐ **Insertion:**

The healthcare professional gently inserts their finger into the rectum. They will feel the back wall of the rectum and then locate the prostate gland, which is situated just in front of the rectum.

☐ **Assessment:**

By moving the finger carefully, the healthcare professional can evaluate the size, shape, and texture of the prostate gland. They check for any abnormalities, such as lumps, nodules, or hard areas.

Purpose:

The primary purpose of a DRE is to help identify any potential abnormalities in the prostate gland that may indicate prostate cancer or other prostate conditions, such as prostatitis or benign prostatic hyperplasia (BPH). It provides valuable information that can contribute to the overall assessment of a patient's prostate health.

Limitations as a screening tool:

☐ **Limited detection:**
A DRE alone is not highly sensitive for detecting early-stage prostate cancer. Small tumors or tumors located in specific areas of the prostate may not be detectable through this method. As a result, relying solely on a DRE for prostate cancer screening may lead to missed diagnoses.

☐ **Operator dependence:**
The accuracy of a DRE can vary depending on the experience and skill of the healthcare professional performing the examination. Factors like size and positioning of the prostate gland can affect the detection of abnormalities, and different healthcare providers may interpret the findings differently.

☐ **False positives and false negatives:**
DRE can sometimes yield false-positive results, suggesting the presence of cancer when none exists. Conversely, false-

negative results can occur, where a cancerous growth is missed during the examination. This highlights the importance of using additional screening methods alongside DRE, such as prostate-specific antigen (PSA) blood tests or imaging techniques like ultrasound or MRI.

- ☐ **Discomfort and patient reluctance:** DRE can be uncomfortable or embarrassing for some individuals, leading to reluctance in undergoing the examination. This may hinder compliance with regular screening, resulting in missed opportunities for early detection.

In summary, while a digital rectal examination plays a role in the diagnosis of prostate cancer by providing important information about the prostate gland, it is not sufficient as a sole screening tool. It should be complemented with other tests, such as PSA blood tests and imaging, to improve the accuracy of detecting prostate cancer at an early stage. Regular discussions with healthcare professionals can help determine the most appropriate screening approach based on an individual's risk factors and preferences.

Imaging Techniques

Transrectal Ultrasound (TRUS):
- **Advantages:**
  - Cost-effective and widely available.
  - Real-time imaging allows for the visualization of the prostate and surrounding structures.
  - Helps guide biopsy procedures by targeting specific areas of concern.
  - Provides information on prostate size, shape, and potential abnormalities.

- **Limitations:**
  - Limited soft tissue contrast, making it challenging to differentiate between benign and malignant tissues.

- o Operator dependence, as image quality and interpretation can vary.
  - o Inability to detect small lesions or assess the spread of cancer beyond the prostate.

- ☐ **Specific Applications:**
  - o Initial evaluation of prostate abnormalities.
  - o Guiding prostate biopsy procedures.
  - o Monitoring disease progression and treatment response.

Magnetic Resonance Imaging (MRI):
- ☐ **Advantages:**
  - o Superior soft tissue contrast, enabling better visualization and differentiation of benign and malignant tissues.
  - o Multi-parametric MRI techniques, such as diffusion-weighted imaging (DWI) and dynamic contrast-enhanced MRI (DCE-MRI), provide additional functional information.

- Improved accuracy in detecting and localizing prostate tumors, including small lesions.
- Evaluation of extracapsular extension, seminal vesicle invasion, and lymph node involvement.

☐ Limitations:
- Higher cost compared to TRUS.
- Limited availability in some regions.
- Susceptible to motion artifacts, requiring patient cooperation and breath-holding techniques.
- False-positive findings may occur, leading to unnecessary biopsies or interventions.

☐ Specific Applications:
- Detection and localization of prostate cancer.
- Assessing tumor aggressiveness and staging.
- Monitoring disease progression and treatment response.

- o Guiding targeted biopsies and focal therapy.

Positron Emission Tomography (PET):
- □ **Advantages:**
    - o Allows for whole-body imaging, facilitating the detection and staging of metastatic disease.
    - o Different radiotracers can provide specific information about tumor metabolism, proliferation, and receptor expression.
    - o PET/CT or PET/MRI fusion images provide anatomical and functional information in combination.

- □ **Limitations:**
    - o Limited sensitivity for small lesions and low-grade tumors.
    - o Availability of specific radiotracers may be limited.
    - o Higher cost compared to other imaging modalities.

- o False-positive findings can occur due to various physiological processes or inflammation.

□ **Specific Applications:**
  - o Staging and restaging of prostate cancer.
  - o Detection of metastatic disease.
  - o Assessment of treatment response and recurrent disease.
  - o Evaluating the aggressiveness of tumors using radiotracers like 18F-choline or 68Ga-PSMA.

It's important to note that the specific applications and limitations can vary depending on the clinical context, availability of resources, and advancements in imaging technology. Consulting with a medical professional is recommended for accurate and up-to-date information on the use of imaging modalities for prostate cancer diagnosis.

Biopsy

Prostate biopsy plays a crucial role in confirming the presence of prostate cancer. It is a procedure in which small tissue samples are collected from the prostate gland to be examined under a microscope by a pathologist. The analysis of these tissue samples provides valuable information about the presence, stage, and grade of prostate cancer.

There are two commonly used techniques for performing a prostate biopsy: transrectal ultrasound-guided biopsy (TRUS biopsy) and transperineal biopsy.

- **Transrectal Ultrasound-Guided Biopsy (TRUS Biopsy):**
  TRUS biopsy is the most common technique used for prostate biopsies. During this procedure, a small ultrasound probe is inserted into the rectum to visualize the prostate gland. The ultrasound images help guide the urologist in targeting specific areas of suspicion within the prostate. Then, a biopsy needle is inserted through the

rectum, and multiple tissue samples are collected from different areas of the prostate. These samples are sent to a pathology laboratory for analysis.

☐ **Transperineal Biopsy:**
Transperineal biopsy involves accessing the prostate gland through the perineum, the area between the scrotum and anus. This technique is typically performed under general or local anesthesia. A biopsy needle is inserted through the perineum to collect tissue samples from the prostate. Transperineal biopsy is often used when TRUS biopsy is challenging or when a more extensive sampling is required. It may also be used in cases where previous biopsy results were negative, but there is still suspicion of prostate cancer.

The importance of pathology analysis cannot be overstated in determining the stage and grade of prostate cancer. Once the biopsy samples are collected, they are sent to a pathology laboratory, where a pathologist examines them under a microscope. The pathologist assesses the tissue for the presence of cancer cells and determines the cancer's grade and stage.

- **Cancer Grade:**
  The grade of prostate cancer is determined by assessing the appearance of cancer cells under a microscope. The most commonly used grading system is the Gleason grading system, which assigns a score ranging from 6 to 10. The Gleason score helps estimate how aggressive the cancer is. Lower scores (6 or below) indicate less aggressive cancer, while higher scores (7-10) suggest more aggressive cancer.

- **Cancer Stage:**
  The stage of prostate cancer refers to the extent of cancer spread beyond the prostate gland. Staging is crucial in determining appropriate treatment options and predicting the prognosis. The pathologist examines the biopsy samples

to assess whether the cancer has spread beyond the prostate gland and into nearby tissues or distant organs. Staging is often determined using the TNM system, which considers tumor size (T), lymph node involvement (N), and distant metastasis (M).

In summary, a prostate biopsy, whether performed using transrectal ultrasound-guided biopsy or transperineal biopsy, is essential for confirming the presence of prostate cancer. The biopsy samples are then sent for pathology analysis, where the cancer grade and stage are determined. This information is crucial in guiding treatment decisions and predicting the prognosis for individuals with prostate cancer.

Genetic Testing

Prostate cancer is a prevalent form of cancer among men worldwide. While various factors contribute to the development of prostate cancer, including age and family history, genetic mutations have gained significant attention in recent years. Advances in genetic testing have enabled researchers and clinicians to identify specific genetic mutations associated with prostate cancer, offering valuable insights into risk assessment, treatment response prediction, and personalized treatment strategies. Two prominent genetic mutations linked to prostate cancer are BRCA1 and BRCA2.

BRCA1 and BRCA2 are well-known genetic mutations typically associated with an increased risk of breast and ovarian cancers in women. However, emerging evidence suggests that these mutations also play a role in prostate cancer susceptibility. Men with BRCA1 or BRCA2 mutations have a higher risk of developing prostate cancer compared to those without these mutations. Furthermore, individuals with BRCA2 mutations tend to have more aggressive forms of prostate cancer, higher rates of recurrence, and a poorer prognosis.

Genetic testing for BRCA1 and BRCA2 mutations in men with suspected or diagnosed prostate cancer has several clinical implications. Firstly, identifying these mutations in prostate cancer patients can help determine the appropriate management strategies and treatment options. For instance, men with BRCA2 mutations may be candidates for more aggressive treatment approaches due to the higher likelihood of aggressive disease progression.

Additionally, genetic testing for prostate cancer can inform the selection of targeted therapies. PARP inhibitors, a class of drugs that target DNA repair pathways, have shown promising results in treating prostate cancer patients with BRCA1 and BRCA2 mutations. Clinical trials have demonstrated that PARP inhibitors can effectively inhibit cancer growth and improve outcomes in this specific subset of patients. Thus, genetic testing allows for a more precise selection of treatment options, potentially leading to better response rates and improved patient outcomes.

Moreover, genetic testing for prostate cancer can have implications for the broader management of patients and their families. Identifying BRCA1 or BRCA2 mutations in prostate cancer patients may warrant further evaluation of family members for these mutations. This information can help identify individuals at increased risk for prostate cancer and other associated cancers, facilitating early detection and preventive measures.

While the field of genetic testing for prostate cancer is still evolving, it holds great potential for improving risk assessment, treatment decision-making, and patient outcomes. As genetic testing technologies continue to advance, more genetic mutations and markers associated with prostate cancer risk and treatment response are likely to be identified. This ongoing research will enable the development of more comprehensive genetic testing panels to enhance personalized treatment strategies and improve overall prostate cancer management.

CHAPTER FIVE

TREATMENTS FOR PROSTATE CANCER AND THEIR SIDE EFFECTS

Prostate cancer is a prevalent form of cancer that affects the prostate gland, a small organ located below the bladder and in front of the rectum in men. It is one of the most common cancers diagnosed in men worldwide. While the term "cure" in the context of cancer can be complex, I will explain the various treatment options available for prostate cancer and discuss the potential for achieving remission or long-term control of the disease.

Prostate cancer treatment depends on several factors, including the stage of the cancer, the aggressiveness of the tumor, the patient's overall health, and their preferences. The primary treatment modalities for prostate cancer include surgery, radiation therapy, hormone therapy, chemotherapy, and immunotherapy. Additionally, active surveillance may be appropriate for some patients with low-risk tumors that are unlikely to progress rapidly.

Surgery Process

Surgery is a common and effective treatment option for prostate cancer, particularly in the early stages of the disease. The primary surgical procedure used for prostate cancer is called a radical prostatectomy, which involves the complete removal of the prostate gland along with some surrounding tissue. This procedure can be performed through open surgery or minimally invasive techniques such as laparoscopic or robotic-assisted surgery. In this explanation, we will explore the various aspects of surgery as a treatment for prostate cancer and its benefits.

Firstly, surgery aims to remove the cancerous prostate gland from the body. The prostate gland is located just below the bladder and surrounds the urethra, the tube through which urine passes out of the body. By removing the prostate, surgery eliminates the source of cancer cells, effectively treating the disease. It is important to note that surgery is typically recommended for localized prostate cancer, where the tumor is confined to the prostate gland and has not spread to other parts of the body.

One of the primary benefits of surgery is the potential for a complete cure. If the cancer is localized, surgery can remove all cancerous cells from the body, effectively eradicating the disease. This can provide patients with a high chance of long-term survival and a potential return to a cancer-free life. However, it is important to note that the success of surgery depends on various factors such as the stage and aggressiveness of the cancer, as well as the patient's overall health.

The choice of surgical approach depends on several factors, including the surgeon's expertise, patient preferences, and the specific characteristics of the cancer. Open surgery involves making an incision in the lower abdomen to access and remove the prostate gland. It allows for direct visualization and manual dexterity, but it typically requires a longer hospital stay and recovery time.

Minimally invasive techniques, such as laparoscopic or robotic-assisted surgery, have gained popularity in recent years. These approaches involve using small incisions and specialized instruments, including a robotic system controlled by the surgeon, to perform the procedure. Robotic-assisted surgery offers several advantages, including improved visualization, enhanced precision, and reduced invasiveness. It allows for greater maneuverability and flexibility, enabling surgeons to perform complex tasks with enhanced precision. Additionally, robotic surgery often results in less blood loss, shorter hospital stays, faster recovery, and reduced post-operative pain compared to open surgery.

During surgery, the surgeon carefully removes the prostate gland, ensuring to remove all cancerous tissue while sparing surrounding healthy tissues to the best extent possible. The nearby lymph nodes may also be sampled or removed to determine if the cancer has spread beyond the prostate. This information helps guide further treatment decisions and prognosis.

In addition to removing the prostate, surgical techniques aim to preserve urinary and sexual functions as much as possible. However, it is important to note that these functions can be affected by the surgery, and there may be temporary or permanent side effects.

Urinary incontinence, the inability to control urine flow, is a potential side effect of surgery. This can occur due to disruption of the urinary sphincter muscles during the procedure. However, advancements in surgical techniques, such as nerve-sparing approaches, have significantly reduced the risk of urinary incontinence. Additionally, post-operative exercises and physical therapy can aid in the recovery of urinary control.

Another potential side effect is erectile dysfunction, the inability to achieve or maintain an erection sufficient for sexual intercourse. The nerves that control erectile function are in close proximity to the prostate gland, and their preservation during surgery is crucial. Surgeons strive to spare these nerves whenever possible to preserve erectile function. However, there is still a risk of temporary or permanent erectile dysfunction following surgery. In some cases, additional treatments such as medications, penile rehabilitation programs, or other interventions may be recommended to help restore sexual function.

Radiation Therapy

Radiation therapy is a widely used and effective treatment option for prostate cancer. It involves the use of high-energy radiation to destroy cancer cells or prevent their growth. Radiation therapy can be delivered externally or internally, depending on the specific characteristics of the cancer and the patient's individual circumstances. In this explanation, we will explore the various aspects of radiation therapy as a treatment for prostate cancer and its benefits.

External beam radiation therapy (EBRT) is the most common form of radiation therapy for prostate cancer. It involves using a machine called a linear accelerator to deliver radiation to the prostate gland from outside the body. Before the treatment begins, detailed imaging, such as computed tomography (CT) scans or magnetic resonance imaging (MRI), is used to precisely map the prostate's position and shape. This allows the radiation oncologist to accurately target the cancer while minimizing exposure to surrounding healthy tissues.

One of the primary benefits of external beam radiation therapy is its non-invasive nature. It does not require any incisions or surgical procedures, making it an attractive option for patients who may not be suitable candidates for surgery or prefer a non-surgical approach. It is also an outpatient procedure, meaning that patients can receive treatment and return home the same day, without the need for hospitalization.

External beam radiation therapy is typically delivered in multiple sessions called fractions over several weeks. Each treatment session lasts a few minutes, and patients typically receive treatments five days a week. This fractionation allows the delivery of effective doses of radiation to the cancer while minimizing damage to surrounding healthy tissues. The total number of treatments depends on various factors, including the stage and aggressiveness of the cancer, as well as the patient's overall health.

Another form of radiation therapy for prostate cancer is brachytherapy, also known as internal radiation therapy. Brachytherapy involves placing tiny radioactive seeds directly into the prostate gland. These seeds emit radiation that destroys the cancer cells over time. Brachytherapy can be delivered in two ways: low-dose rate (LDR) and high-dose rate (HDR).

In LDR brachytherapy, small radioactive seeds, about the size of a grain of rice, are permanently implanted into the prostate gland. The seeds release low-dose radiation continuously over several months, gradually destroying the cancer cells. Over time, the radioactivity of the seeds decreases, and they remain in the prostate gland without causing any harm.

HDR brachytherapy, on the other hand, involves placing temporary radioactive sources into the prostate gland for a short period, typically a few minutes. These sources emit high-dose radiation, and the treatment is carefully planned and delivered in multiple sessions. After each session, the radioactive sources are removed, and no radioactivity remains in the body between treatments.

Brachytherapy offers several advantages. Firstly, it allows for a high dose of radiation to be delivered directly to the prostate gland while minimizing exposure to surrounding healthy tissues. This targeted approach can result in effective cancer control with fewer side effects. Additionally, brachytherapy is a convenient treatment option, as it is usually completed within a day or a few sessions, unlike external beam radiation therapy, which requires multiple weeks of treatment.

Radiation therapy works by damaging the DNA within cancer cells, preventing them from dividing and growing. The damaged cancer cells are then either eliminated by the body's natural defense mechanisms or undergo programmed cell death, known as apoptosis. Radiation therapy affects both cancerous and healthy cells, but healthy cells have a greater ability to repair themselves. Therefore, the goal of radiation therapy is to deliver enough radiation to the cancer cells while minimizing the impact on healthy tissues.

Radiation therapy can be curative for localized prostate cancer, particularly in cases where surgery may not be feasible or preferred.

Hormone Therapy

Hormone therapy, also known as androgen deprivation therapy (ADT), is a systemic treatment approach used in the management of prostate cancer. It involves suppressing or blocking the production or action of male hormones, particularly testosterone, which plays a crucial role in the growth and development of prostate cancer cells. Hormone therapy can be an effective treatment option for both localized and advanced prostate cancer. In this explanation, we will explore the various aspects of hormone therapy as a treatment for prostate cancer and its benefits.

Prostate cancer cells are dependent on androgens, including testosterone, for their growth and survival. By reducing the levels of androgens or blocking their action, hormone therapy aims to inhibit the growth and spread of prostate cancer cells. This treatment approach is based on the understanding that prostate cancer is an androgen-dependent disease, and manipulating the hormonal environment can significantly impact the progression of the cancer.

Hormone therapy can be administered through different methods, including medications that either reduce the production of androgens in the body or block their action on cancer cells. The choice of hormone therapy depends on various factors, such as the stage of the cancer, the aggressiveness of the tumor, and the overall health of the patient.

One of the primary goals of hormone therapy is to achieve and maintain a low level of testosterone in the body. This can be accomplished through medications known as luteinizing hormone-releasing hormone (LHRH) agonists or antagonists. LHRH agonists work by initially stimulating the production of luteinizing hormone (LH), which in turn stimulates the testicles to produce testosterone. However, with continuous use, these medications desensitize the receptors in the pituitary gland, leading to a decrease in LH production and a subsequent reduction in testosterone levels. LHRH antagonists, on the other hand, directly block the receptors in the pituitary gland, resulting in an immediate decrease in testosterone production.

Another medication commonly used in hormone therapy is an anti-androgen. Anti-androgens work by blocking the action of androgens on prostate cancer cells. They can be used in combination with LHRH agonists or antagonists to maximize the suppression of androgens. Anti-androgens can either be non-steroidal, such as bicalutamide and flutamide, or steroidal, such as cyproterone acetate.

In addition to medications that reduce androgen production or block their action, there are other strategies to achieve hormonal suppression. For example, surgical removal of the testicles, known as orchiectomy, can be performed to eliminate the primary source of testosterone production. Orchiectomy provides a permanent reduction in testosterone levels and is often considered in cases where long-term hormone therapy is required.

Hormone therapy can be used at different stages of prostate cancer treatment. In localized prostate cancer, hormone therapy may be used as a neoadjuvant treatment before other interventions, such as radiation therapy or surgery. By reducing the size of the tumor and inhibiting its growth, hormone therapy can make these treatments more effective. It can also be used as an adjuvant treatment after surgery or radiation therapy to further suppress any remaining cancer cells and reduce the risk of recurrence.

In advanced or metastatic prostate cancer, hormone therapy is often the primary treatment. It is used to control the growth and spread of cancer cells, relieve symptoms, and prolong survival. While hormone therapy is not curative in advanced prostate cancer, it can significantly slow down the progression of the disease and improve the quality of life.

Hormone therapy has several benefits as a treatment for prostate cancer. It can shrink the size of the prostate tumor, relieve symptoms associated with the disease, and slow down the growth of cancer cells. In some cases, hormone therapy can lead to long-term remission and control of the disease. However, it is important to note that hormone therapy is not a cure for prostate cancer, particularly in advanced or metastatic stages. Over time, prostate cancer cells may develop resistance to hormone therapy, leading to a progression of the disease.

The effectiveness of hormone therapy varies depending on the individual and the characteristics of the cancer. While hormone therapy can initially cause a significant reduction in prostate-specific antigen (PSA) levels, which is a marker for prostate cancer activity, the cancer cells may eventually adapt and become resistant to hormonal suppression. This is known as castration-resistant prostate cancer (CRPC) or hormone-resistant prostate cancer.

When prostate cancer becomes resistant to hormone therapy, additional treatment options may be considered. These may include chemotherapy, immunotherapy, targeted therapies, or participation in clinical trials investigating new treatment approaches. It is important for patients and their healthcare providers to discuss the available options and develop a personalized treatment plan based on the specific circumstances of the disease.

Hormone therapy can have side effects that impact a patient's quality of life. The reduction in testosterone levels can cause a range of physical and emotional changes. Some common side effects of hormone therapy include hot flashes, decreased sexual desire, erectile dysfunction, fatigue, weight gain, loss of muscle mass, and changes in mood. These side effects can vary in severity and may have a significant impact on a patient's well-being.

Management of the side effects of hormone therapy is an essential part of the treatment process. Healthcare providers can offer strategies to alleviate the symptoms and provide support. For example, medications can be prescribed to manage hot flashes or address sexual dysfunction. Lifestyle modifications, such as regular exercise and a healthy diet, can help mitigate some of the side effects, such as weight gain and fatigue.

It is crucial for patients undergoing hormone therapy to maintain regular communication with their healthcare team. Monitoring PSA levels and conducting regular follow-up appointments are necessary to evaluate the response to treatment and make any necessary adjustments. The healthcare team can also provide support and guidance throughout the treatment process, addressing any concerns or questions that may arise.

In summary, hormone therapy is a solid treatment option for prostate cancer, particularly in localized and advanced stages of the disease. It works by reducing the levels of androgens, primarily testosterone, to inhibit the growth and spread of prostate cancer cells. Hormone therapy can provide significant benefits, including tumor shrinkage, symptom relief, and improved overall survival. However, it is not a cure for prostate cancer, and resistance to hormonal suppression may develop over time. Close monitoring and regular communication with healthcare providers are essential to optimize the effectiveness of hormone therapy and manage any side effects that may arise.

Chemotherapy

Chemotherapy is a systemic treatment option for prostate cancer that uses medications to destroy cancer cells or inhibit their growth. It is typically used in advanced stages of the disease when the cancer has spread beyond the prostate gland or has become resistant to hormone therapy. In this explanation, we will explore the various aspects of chemotherapy as a treatment for prostate cancer and its benefits.

Chemotherapy drugs are designed to target and kill rapidly dividing cells, including cancer cells. Unlike localized treatments such as surgery or radiation therapy, chemotherapy works throughout the body, reaching cancer cells that may have spread to distant sites. The drugs are administered either intravenously or orally and circulate through the bloodstream, targeting cancer cells wherever they may be.

Chemotherapy for prostate cancer typically involves a combination of drugs, each with its own mechanism of action and potential side effects. The specific combination and dosage of chemotherapy drugs depend on various factors, including the stage of the cancer, the patient's overall health, and any prior treatments received.

One of the primary goals of chemotherapy in prostate cancer is to slow down the progression of the disease, alleviate symptoms, and prolong survival. While chemotherapy is not considered curative for advanced prostate cancer, it can significantly impact the course of the disease and improve the quality of life for patients.

Chemotherapy can be used as the primary treatment for metastatic prostate cancer, particularly in cases where the cancer has spread to distant organs such as the bones or lymph nodes. It aims to control the growth and spread of cancer cells, shrink tumors, and alleviate symptoms associated with the disease.

Additionally, chemotherapy may be used in combination with hormone therapy for certain patients. This approach, known as combined or dual therapy, combines the benefits of both treatments to maximize the effectiveness of prostate cancer treatment. By combining hormone therapy and chemotherapy, the aim is to target cancer cells through multiple mechanisms and increase the chances of disease control.

Chemotherapy can also be used as a salvage treatment option for patients who have experienced a recurrence of prostate cancer after surgery or radiation therapy. In these cases, chemotherapy may be employed to target any remaining cancer cells and prevent further disease progression.

Chemotherapy drugs used in the treatment of prostate cancer include docetaxel, cabazitaxel, and mitoxantrone. These medications work by interfering with the division and growth of cancer cells, ultimately leading to their destruction. These drugs may be used alone or in combination with other chemotherapy agents or targeted therapies.

The administration of chemotherapy is typically done in cycles, with a period of treatment followed by a rest period. This approach allows healthy cells to recover from the effects of chemotherapy while still targeting cancer cells. The length and frequency of chemotherapy cycles depend on the specific drugs used and the patient's response to treatment.

The effectiveness of chemotherapy varies depending on the individual and the characteristics of the cancer. In some cases, chemotherapy can lead to a significant reduction in prostate-specific antigen (PSA) levels, a marker for prostate cancer activity. Decreased PSA levels indicate a response to treatment and may be associated with tumor shrinkage and symptom improvement.

However, it is important to note that not all patients respond to chemotherapy in the same way. Some individuals may experience a partial or complete response to treatment, while others may have stable disease or even disease progression. The response to chemotherapy can be influenced by various factors, including the aggressiveness of the cancer, the presence of specific genetic mutations, and the overall health of the patient.

As with any treatment, chemotherapy can have side effects that impact a patient's quality of life. The drugs used in chemotherapy can affect both cancer cells and healthy cells, leading to a range of side effects. These may include fatigue, nausea, vomiting, hair loss, decreased blood cell counts (resulting in increased susceptibility to infection or bleeding), neuropathy (tingling or numbness in the extremities), loss of appetite, weight changes, diarrhea or constipation, and changes in taste or smell.

Hair loss, or alopecia, is another potential side effect of chemotherapy. This can be emotionally distressing for many patients, as hair loss is often associated with changes in appearance and self-image. It is important for patients to discuss the possibility of hair loss with their healthcare team and explore options such as scalp cooling or wigs to help manage this aspect of treatment.

Chemotherapy drugs can also affect the bone marrow, leading to decreased blood cell counts. This can result in an increased risk of infection, bleeding, and anemia. Regular blood tests are conducted during chemotherapy to monitor blood cell counts, and adjustments to the treatment regimen may be made if necessary.

Patients should report any signs of infection, such as fever or persistent cough, as well as any unusual bleeding or bruising to their healthcare provider.

Neuropathy, or damage to the nerves, is another potential side effect of chemotherapy. It can manifest as tingling or numbness in the extremities, such as the hands and feet. In some cases, it may cause pain or difficulty with fine motor skills. Patients should inform their healthcare team if they experience any symptoms of neuropathy, as adjustments to the treatment regimen or additional medications may be necessary to manage this side effect.

Managing the side effects of chemotherapy is an essential part of the treatment process. Open and honest communication with the healthcare team is crucial, as they can provide guidance, prescribe medications, and recommend strategies to alleviate and manage side effects. It is important for patients to report any new or worsening symptoms promptly, as timely intervention can often prevent or minimize the impact of side effects.

In conclusion, chemotherapy is a solid treatment option for prostate cancer, particularly in advanced stages of the disease. It works by targeting cancer cells throughout the body, aiming to slow down disease progression, alleviate symptoms, and improve overall survival. Chemotherapy can be used as the primary treatment for metastatic prostate cancer or in combination with other therapies. However, it is important to note that chemotherapy is not curative and may have side effects that impact a patient's quality of life. The side effects vary from person to person and can include fatigue, nausea, hair loss, decreased blood cell counts, neuropathy, changes in appetite and weight, and changes in taste or smell. Close collaboration with the healthcare team is crucial to manage these side effects effectively and optimize treatment outcomes.

Immunotherapy

Immunotherapy is an innovative treatment approach that harnesses the power of the immune system to fight cancer. It has emerged as a promising treatment option for various types of cancer, including prostate cancer. In this explanation, we will explore the concept of immunotherapy and its application in the treatment of prostate cancer.

The immune system is a complex network of cells, tissues, and organs that work together to defend the body against foreign invaders, such as bacteria and viruses. It also plays a crucial role in recognizing and eliminating abnormal or cancerous cells. However, cancer cells can develop mechanisms to evade the immune system's surveillance, allowing them to grow and spread.

Immunotherapy aims to enhance the body's immune response against cancer cells by either boosting the immune system or removing the barriers that prevent the immune system from effectively targeting cancer cells. There are different types of immunotherapy approaches used in the treatment of prostate cancer, including immune checkpoint inhibitors, therapeutic vaccines, and adoptive cell therapies.

One of the most widely studied forms of immunotherapy in prostate cancer is immune checkpoint inhibitors. Immune checkpoints are molecules present on immune cells that regulate the intensity and duration of immune responses. Cancer cells can hijack these checkpoints to evade immune attack. Checkpoint inhibitors block these checkpoints, enabling the immune system to mount a more robust and sustained attack against cancer cells.

In prostate cancer, immune checkpoint inhibitors such as pembrolizumab and nivolumab have shown efficacy in a subset of patients with advanced or metastatic disease. These drugs target immune checkpoints like PD-1 (programmed cell death protein 1) or PD-L1 (programmed death-ligand 1), which are often upregulated in cancer cells. By blocking the PD-1/PD-L1 interaction, immune checkpoint inhibitors release the brakes on the immune system, allowing immune cells to recognize and attack cancer cells more effectively.

Clinical trials evaluating immune checkpoint inhibitors in prostate cancer have shown promising results, particularly in patients with advanced disease who have exhausted other treatment options. However, it is important to note that not all patients respond to immune checkpoint inhibitors, and further research is needed to identify biomarkers that can predict treatment response.

Another immunotherapy approach being investigated in prostate cancer is therapeutic vaccines. Unlike traditional vaccines that prevent infections, therapeutic vaccines are designed to stimulate the immune system and train it to recognize and target cancer cells. These vaccines typically contain antigens derived from prostate cancer cells, along with substances that enhance the immune response.

Sipuleucel-T is an example of a therapeutic vaccine approved for the treatment of advanced prostate cancer. It involves collecting a patient's immune cells through a process called leukapheresis, which are then exposed to a prostate cancer antigen known as prostatic acid phosphatase (PAP) and a stimulatory factor called granulocyte-macrophage colony-stimulating factor (GM-CSF). The activated immune cells are then reinfused into the patient, where they can target and attack prostate cancer cells.

Therapeutic vaccines aim to induce a specific immune response against prostate cancer cells, which can lead to tumor shrinkage and improved survival. However, their effectiveness may vary among patients, and more research is needed to optimize their design and identify patient populations that are most likely to benefit.

Adoptive cell therapies are another form of immunotherapy being explored in prostate cancer. These therapies involve modifying a patient's own immune cells, typically T cells, to enhance their ability to recognize and attack cancer cells. One approach is chimeric antigen receptor (CAR) T-cell therapy, where T cells are engineered to express receptors that specifically target prostate cancer antigens.

CAR T-cell therapy has shown promising results in other types of cancer, but its application in prostate cancer is still in the early stages of development. Researchers are actively working on identifying specific prostate cancer antigens that can be targeted by CAR T-cell therapy. Additionally, combination approaches with other treatments, such as immune checkpoint inhibitors or chemotherapy, are being explored to enhance the effectiveness of CAR T-cell therapy in prostate cancer.

Like any treatment, immunotherapy can have side effects, although they tend to differ from those associated with traditional chemotherapy or radiation therapy. Immune-related adverse events (irAEs) can occur as a result of the immune system being activated. These can include inflammation of organs or tissues, skin rashes, diarrhea, liver inflammation, and hormonal imbalances. However, irAEs are typically manageable with close monitoring and appropriate medical intervention.

The selection of patients for immunotherapy and the monitoring of treatment response are important considerations. Biomarkers such as PD-L1 expression, tumor mutational burden, and microsatellite instability can help identify patients who are more likely to respond to immune checkpoint inhibitors. Regular imaging scans and blood tests, including prostate-specific antigen (PSA) levels, are performed to monitor treatment response and disease progression.

It is essential to note that immunotherapy is not a one-size-fits-all approach, and its effectiveness can vary among individuals. Some patients may experience a significant response with durable remission, while others may have stable disease or minimal response. Ongoing research is focused on understanding the factors that influence treatment response and identifying strategies to enhance the effectiveness of immunotherapy in prostate cancer.

In conclusion, immunotherapy is an evolving treatment approach for prostate cancer that harnesses the power of the immune system to target and attack cancer cells. Immune checkpoint inhibitors, therapeutic vaccines, and adoptive cell therapies are among the different immunotherapy strategies being explored in prostate cancer treatment. These approaches hold promise in improving outcomes for patients with advanced or metastatic disease, particularly in those who have limited treatment options. While immunotherapy has shown encouraging results, further research is needed to optimize its use, identify predictive biomarkers, and develop combination approaches to enhance treatment efficacy. Collaboration between researchers, healthcare providers, and patients is crucial to advancing the field of immunotherapy and improving outcomes for individuals with prostate cancer.

Side effects of prostate cancer treatment

Prostate cancer and its treatments can lead to various side effects that can significantly impact a patient's quality of life. The specific side effects experienced can vary depending on factors such as the stage of the cancer, the treatment received, and the individual's overall health. In this explanation, we will explore some of the common side effects associated with prostate cancer and its treatments.

Urinary Problems:

The prostate gland surrounds the urethra, which carries urine from the bladder out of the body. Prostate cancer can cause urinary symptoms such as frequent urination, difficulty starting or stopping urination, weak urine flow, or the sensation of incomplete bladder emptying. These symptoms may be present due to the tumor's location or if it has spread to nearby tissues. Additionally, certain treatments like surgery or radiation therapy can cause temporary or long-term urinary side effects, including urinary incontinence (involuntary leakage of urine) or urinary retention (inability to empty the bladder completely).

Erectile Dysfunction:

Erectile dysfunction (ED) is a common side effect of prostate cancer and its treatments. The nerves and blood vessels that control erections can be affected by the cancer or damaged during surgery or radiation therapy. Hormone therapy, which aims to reduce the levels of testosterone in the body, can also contribute to ED. Depending on the extent of nerve damage or the treatment received, some men may experience temporary or permanent difficulty achieving or maintaining an erection.

Bowel Problems:

Radiation therapy for prostate cancer can lead to bowel-related side effects. The rectum, which is located near the prostate gland, can be exposed to radiation during treatment, resulting in symptoms such as diarrhea, rectal urgency (a sudden and strong urge to have a bowel movement), or rectal bleeding. These side effects are typically temporary and improve over time, but in some cases, they may persist.

Fatigue:

Fatigue is a common side effect experienced by cancer patients, including those with prostate cancer. It is characterized by a persistent feeling of tiredness, lack of energy, and a reduced ability to carry out daily activities. Fatigue can be caused by the cancer itself, as well as treatments such as radiation therapy, chemotherapy, or hormone therapy. Managing fatigue often involves a combination of rest, balanced nutrition, physical activity, and addressing any underlying causes or comorbidities.

Hormonal Changes:

Hormone therapy, also known as androgen deprivation therapy (ADT), is a common treatment for advanced prostate cancer. It works by reducing the levels of testosterone in the body, which can slow down the growth of prostate cancer cells. However, this hormonal manipulation can lead to side effects such as hot flashes, decreased libido (sex drive), loss of muscle mass, weight gain, and mood changes. Some of these side effects may be managed with lifestyle adjustments or medications, but they can still impact a patient's well-being and quality of life.

Psychological and Emotional Impact:

Prostate cancer and its treatments can have a significant psychological and emotional impact on patients. The diagnosis of cancer can evoke feelings of fear, anxiety, depression, or uncertainty about the future. Treatment-related side effects, changes in body image, and sexual dysfunction can also affect a patient's self-esteem and overall emotional well-being. It is important for patients to have access to psychological support, counseling services, or support groups to address these emotional challenges and enhance coping mechanisms.

It is crucial for patients to communicate openly with their healthcare team about any side effects they are experiencing. Healthcare providers can offer strategies to manage and alleviate these side effects, and in some cases, additional medications or interventions may be recommended. Supportive care, which focuses on improving a patient's overall well-being and quality of life, plays a crucial role in addressing side effects and helping patients navigate through their prostate cancer journey.

For urinary problems, healthcare providers may recommend lifestyle modifications such as reducing fluid intake before bedtime, bladder training exercises, or medications to improve urinary function. In cases of erectile dysfunction, treatments such as oral medications, penile injections, vacuum erection devices, or surgical interventions like penile implants may be considered. Healthcare providers can also refer patients to specialists, such as urologists or sexual health counselors, who can provide further guidance and support.

Bowel problems related to radiation therapy can often be managed with dietary adjustments, such as increasing fiber intake or avoiding certain foods that may exacerbate symptoms. Medications may be prescribed to alleviate diarrhea or relieve rectal discomfort. It is important for patients to maintain open communication with their healthcare team to ensure appropriate management of these side effects.

Fatigue can be managed through lifestyle modifications, including regular exercise, balanced nutrition, adequate rest, and stress reduction techniques. Healthcare providers may also address underlying causes of fatigue, such as anemia or hormone imbalances, and recommend appropriate interventions.

Hormonal changes resulting from androgen deprivation therapy can be managed with lifestyle modifications and medications. For example, hot flashes may be alleviated with lifestyle changes such as wearing layered clothing, avoiding triggers like caffeine or spicy foods, or medications that target hot flashes specifically. Changes in mood or emotional well-being can be addressed through counseling, support groups, or referral to mental health professionals.

Psychological support is essential for addressing the psychological and emotional impact of prostate cancer. Healthcare providers can refer patients to psychologists, psychiatrists, or social workers who specialize in oncology and can provide counseling and support services. Support groups, both in-person and online, can connect patients with others going through similar experiences and provide a platform for sharing concerns, emotions, and coping strategies.

In summary, prostate cancer and its treatments can result in various side effects that can impact a patient's quality of life. Open communication with the healthcare team is crucial in managing and addressing these side effects effectively. Healthcare providers can offer strategies, medications, and referrals to supportive care services to help alleviate the physical, emotional, and psychological challenges associated with prostate cancer. Through comprehensive and multidisciplinary care, patients can receive the support they need to navigate their prostate cancer journey with improved well-being and enhanced quality of life.

It is important to note that the term "cure" in cancer treatment can be subjective and dependent on various factors. Prostate cancer can be classified into different stages (from I to IV) and grades (Gleason score), which reflect the aggressiveness and extent of the disease. For localized prostate cancer (stages I and II), curative treatment options such as surgery and radiation therapy have a higher chance of complete remission or long-term control. However, for advanced prostate cancer (stages III and IV), the goal shifts towards managing the disease, prolonging survival, and improving the quality of life.

In addition to these standard treatments, there are also newer treatments being developed for prostate cancer, such as targeted therapy that involves using drugs that specifically target certain proteins or genes that are involved in cancer growth.

In conclusion, prostate cancer can be cured if it is detected early and has not spread beyond the prostate gland. There are several treatment options available, including surgery, radiation therapy, hormone therapy, immunotherapy and chemotherapy, as well as newer treatments such as and targeted therapy. The choice of treatment depends on various factors, and patients should discuss their options with their doctor to determine the best course of action for their specific case. Regular screenings for prostate cancer are recommended for men over 50, or earlier for those with a family history of the disease or other risk factors.

CHAPTER SIX

COPING WITH PROSTATE CANCER

Navigating the Journey to Healing and Resilicnoo

Prostate cancer is a significant health concern affecting millions of men worldwide. Upon receiving a prostate cancer diagnosis, individuals are confronted with numerous challenges physical, emotional, and psychological. Coping with prostate cancer requires a comprehensive approach that encompasses medical treatments, self-care strategies, support systems, and a positive mindset. This essay aims to explore various aspects of coping with prostate cancer, providing insights into essential coping mechanisms, empowering individuals to navigate the journey towards healing and resilience.

Understanding Prostate Cancer:

Prostate cancer originates in the prostate gland, a crucial part of the male reproductive system. Understanding the nature of prostate cancer is pivotal in coping with the condition effectively. Prostate cancer is typically categorized based on the severity of the disease, including stages and grades, which influence treatment decisions. Patients and their families must educate themselves about the different treatment options available, including surgery, radiation therapy, hormone therapy, and active surveillance, to make informed decisions tailored to their specific situation.

Emotional and Psychological Coping:

A prostate cancer diagnosis often triggers a range of emotions, including fear, anxiety, sadness, and anger. Emotional and psychological coping strategies are essential in maintaining overall well-being throughout the treatment process. Expressing emotions openly and seeking support from loved ones or joining support groups can provide an outlet for emotional release and foster a sense of belonging. Additionally, engaging in relaxation techniques, such as deep breathing exercises, meditation, and mindfulness practices, can help alleviate stress and promote emotional resilience.

Building a Support Network:

Creating a support network is vital for individuals coping with prostate cancer. This network may consist of family members, friends, healthcare professionals, and support groups specifically tailored to prostate cancer patients. Sharing experiences, fears, and triumphs with others facing similar challenges can provide a sense of solidarity and alleviate feelings of isolation. Moreover, professional counseling or therapy can offer valuable tools to cope with emotional distress, strengthen coping skills, and promote a positive outlook.

Self-Care and Lifestyle Changes:

Self-care plays a critical role in coping with prostate cancer. Making positive lifestyle changes, such as adopting a balanced diet rich in fruits, vegetables, and whole grains, can boost overall health and strengthen the body's ability to fight cancer. Regular exercise, tailored to individual capabilities, can improve physical strength, reduce treatment side effects, and enhance emotional well-being. Adequate sleep, managing stress levels, and avoiding tobacco and excessive alcohol consumption are additional self-care practices that can contribute to coping effectively with prostate cancer.

Managing Treatment Side Effects:

Prostate cancer treatments often come with side effects that can affect quality of life. Understanding and managing these side effects is essential for coping successfully. Common side effects include urinary incontinence, erectile dysfunction, fatigue, and hormonal changes. Open communication with healthcare providers is crucial to address these concerns promptly. Patients can benefit from specialized interventions, such as pelvic floor exercises, medications, and lifestyle adjustments, to mitigate treatment-related challenges.

Positive Mindset and Resilience:

Maintaining a positive mindset can significantly impact the coping process. Developing resilience—the ability to adapt and bounce back from adversity—is key to navigating the challenges of prostate cancer. Fostering a positive outlook involves reframing negative thoughts, setting realistic goals, celebrating small victories, and maintaining hope. Engaging in activities that bring joy and purpose, such as hobbies, volunteering, or spending time with loved ones, can uplift spirits and enhance overall well-being.

Navigating Survivorship:

For many prostate cancer survivors, the journey does not end with treatment completion. Navigating survivorship involves adapting to a "new normal" and addressing the physical, emotional, and practical challenges that may arise. Regular follow-up visits, continued self-care practices, and monitoring for potential recurrence are essential. Emotional support and counseling remain crucial during this phase, as survivors may face fear of recurrence, anxiety, depression, or concerns about their future health. Engaging in survivorship programs and connecting with other survivors can provide a sense of community and shared experiences, facilitating the transition into the post-treatment phase.

Open Communication and Shared Decision-Making:

Throughout the prostate cancer journey, open and honest communication with healthcare providers is vital. Engaging in shared decision-making empowers individuals to actively participate in their treatment plans, express their preferences, and ask questions. Understanding the risks, benefits, and potential outcomes of different treatment options enables patients to make informed decisions aligned with their values and goals. Effective communication fosters trust, reduces anxiety, and ensures a collaborative approach to managing prostate cancer.

Educating Oneself and Loved Ones:

Prostate cancer can affect not only the individual diagnosed but also their loved ones. Education about the disease, treatment options, and coping strategies is essential for both patients and their support system. By learning together, individuals can better understand the challenges, offer support, and actively participate in the recovery process. Knowledge empowers individuals to ask informed questions, seek appropriate resources, and make lifestyle adjustments that promote overall well-being for everyone involved.

Advocacy and Support for Prostate Cancer Research:

Coping with prostate cancer extends beyond personal experiences. Advocacy for prostate cancer research and support for organizations dedicated to advancing knowledge and treatment options are crucial in improving outcomes for future generations. Engaging in awareness campaigns, fundraising events, and community initiatives not only contributes to the fight against prostate cancer but also provides a sense of purpose and empowerment for individuals coping with the disease.

Coping with prostate cancer is a multifaceted journey that requires comprehensive strategies encompassing physical, emotional, and psychological well-being. Understanding the nature of the disease, building a strong support network, practicing self-care, managing treatment side effects, and fostering a positive mindset are essential elements of coping effectively. Navigating survivorship and advocating for prostate cancer research further enhance the journey towards healing and resilience. By implementing these coping mechanisms, individuals can not only endure the challenges of prostate cancer but also thrive, leading fulfilling lives beyond their diagnosis.

CHAPTER SEVEN

PREVENTION OF PROSTATE CANCER

Lifestyle Changes

Lifestyle changes such as regular exercise, a healthy diet, and weight management can help prevent prostate cancer. Studies have shown that men who maintain a healthy weight and eat a diet high in fruits, vegetables, and whole grains have a lower risk of developing prostate cancer.

In recent years, lifestyle changes have gained attention as potential interventions to reduce the risk of prostate cancer. This article delves into the impact of three key lifestyle changes: regular exercise, a healthy diet, and weight management. By examining the scientific evidence and underlying mechanisms, we can gain a comprehensive understanding of how these lifestyle modifications can contribute to the prevention of prostate cancer.

Regular physical activity has been associated with numerous health benefits, including a potential protective effect against prostate cancer. Studies have consistently demonstrated an inverse relationship between exercise and prostate cancer risk. Engaging in moderate to vigorous physical activity, such as brisk walking, jogging, or swimming, can significantly reduce the risk of developing prostate cancer. The underlying mechanisms through which exercise exerts its protective effects involve hormonal modulation, improved immune function, inflammation reduction, and enhanced DNA repair capacity.

Adopting a healthy diet rich in fruits, vegetables, whole grains, and lean proteins has been associated with a lower risk of prostate cancer. Several dietary factors have demonstrated protective effects against prostate cancer, such as lycopene, selenium, cruciferous vegetables, and omega-3 fatty acids. These components possess antioxidant, anti-inflammatory, and anti-carcinogenic properties, which help to mitigate the development and progression of prostate cancer. Additionally, reducing the intake of processed foods, red meat, and high-fat dairy products has been linked to a decreased risk of prostate cancer.

Maintaining a healthy weight is crucial for reducing the risk of prostate cancer. Obesity and excess body fat have been associated with an increased risk of aggressive prostate cancer and disease progression. Adipose tissue produces hormones and cytokines that can promote inflammation and hormonal imbalances, contributing to prostate cancer development. By adopting weight management strategies, such as portion control, regular physical activity, and a balanced diet, individuals can significantly reduce their risk of developing prostate cancer.

Lifestyle changes play a critical role in the prevention of prostate cancer. Regular exercise, a healthy diet, and weight management have been consistently associated with a decreased risk of prostate cancer development. Engaging in regular physical activity helps to modulate hormonal levels, bolster immune function, and reduce inflammation, all of which contribute to the prevention of prostate cancer. A healthy diet, rich in fruits, vegetables, and lean proteins, provides essential nutrients and bioactive compounds that possess anti-carcinogenic properties. Additionally, weight management helps to reduce the production of adipose tissue-derived hormones and cytokines that can fuel prostate cancer growth. By adopting these lifestyle changes, men can take proactive steps to reduce their risk of prostate cancer and improve their overall health. Further research and public health initiatives are essential to raise awareness and promote the adoption of these lifestyle modifications on a global scale.

Screening and Early Detection

Early detection plays a pivotal role in ensuring successful treatment outcomes. Screening tests, such as the prostate-specific antigen (PSA) test, have been instrumental in identifying prostate cancer at its earliest stages, often before symptoms manifest. This article explores the significance of screening and early detection in prostate cancer prevention, particularly for individuals at high risk. By understanding the benefits, limitations, and considerations surrounding prostate cancer screening, men can make informed decisions and proactively engage in discussions with healthcare professionals to establish suitable screening strategies.

Screening for prostate cancer involves the use of tests to detect the disease in asymptomatic individuals. The PSA test, a blood test that measures levels of prostate-specific antigen, is the most widely employed screening tool. Early detection enables timely intervention, leading to improved treatment outcomes and reduced mortality rates. Regular screening can detect prostate cancer at its earliest stages, when treatment options are more diverse and effective. Moreover, identifying aggressive forms of prostate cancer early allows for tailored treatment plans, minimizing the risk of disease progression and metastasis.

While screening has notable benefits, there are several considerations to bear in mind. The PSA test has limitations, such as false-positive results, leading to unnecessary biopsies and potential overdiagnosis. The test may also yield false-negative results, providing false reassurance. Additionally, the controversy surrounding the optimal PSA threshold for further investigation has prompted ongoing debate and research. Factors like age, race, family history, and individual risk profiles must be considered when determining the need for screening and establishing appropriate thresholds.

Certain populations face a higher risk of developing prostate cancer due to factors such as age, race, and family history. Men with a family history of prostate cancer, particularly those with affected first-degree relatives, are considered at elevated risk. For these individuals, initiating discussions with healthcare providers about screening options is vital. Guidelines may recommend earlier and more frequent screening for high-risk individuals, allowing for timely detection and intervention.

Shared decision-making between patients and healthcare professionals is crucial when considering prostate cancer screening. Healthcare providers should engage in comprehensive discussions about the benefits, limitations, potential risks, and uncertainties associated with screening. Patient education plays a pivotal role in enabling individuals to make informed choices aligned with their values, preferences, and risk profiles. Understanding the potential benefits and drawbacks of screening empowers men to actively participate in their healthcare decisions.

Early detection through screening tests, notably the PSA test, is integral to prostate cancer prevention. Despite considerations surrounding false-positive and false-negative results, appropriate screening can significantly contribute to improved treatment outcomes and reduced mortality rates. Men at high risk, including those with a family history of prostate cancer, should engage in discussions with healthcare providers to determine suitable screening options and schedules. By embracing shared decision-making and informed choices, individuals can navigate the complexities of prostate cancer screening, ensuring early detection and timely interventions that can ultimately save lives.

Chemoprevention

Chemoprevention, a preventive approach involving the use of drugs and substances, holds promise in reducing the risk of developing and progressing prostate cancer. This article examines the role of chemoprevention in prostate cancer prevention, focusing on specific drugs and substances that have shown potential in scientific studies. Notably, finasteride and dutasteride, medications primarily used for benign prostatic hyperplasia, have demonstrated effectiveness in lowering the risk of prostate cancer. Additionally, natural compounds such as green tea and lycopene have garnered attention for their potential chemopreventive properties. Understanding the current research and mechanisms underlying chemoprevention can contribute to informed decisions and future advancements in prostate cancer prevention.

Finasteride and dutasteride, both 5-alpha-reductase inhibitors, have been extensively studied for their chemopreventive effects on prostate cancer. These medications reduce levels of dihydrotestosterone (DHT), a hormone implicated in the development and growth of prostate cancer. Clinical trials, such as the Prostate Cancer Prevention Trial (PCPT), demonstrated that finasteride reduced the incidence of prostate cancer by approximately 25% in men at average risk. Dutasteride has shown similar effectiveness in lowering the risk of prostate cancer development. However, it is essential to consider potential side effects and weigh the benefits and risks of these medications before use.

Green tea, rich in polyphenols and catechins, has gained attention for its potential chemopreventive properties against various cancers, including prostate cancer. The compounds found in green tea possess antioxidant, anti-inflammatory, and anti-carcinogenic properties that may inhibit the growth and spread of prostate cancer cells. While research on green tea and prostate cancer is still evolving, several studies have shown promising results, suggesting a potential protective effect. However, the optimal dosage and duration of green tea consumption for chemoprevention require further investigation.

Lycopene, a carotenoid pigment found in tomatoes and other red fruits, has been studied for its potential role in prostate cancer prevention. This natural compound exhibits antioxidant and anti-inflammatory properties that may help inhibit the development and progression of prostate cancer cells. Some epidemiological studies have suggested an inverse relationship between lycopene intake and prostate cancer risk. However, clinical trial results have been mixed, highlighting the need for further research to elucidate the optimal dosage, bioavailability, and potential interactions with other compounds.

Beyond finasteride, dutasteride, green tea, and lycopene, ongoing research explores other drugs and substances for their chemopreventive potential against prostate cancer. These include nonsteroidal anti-inflammatory drugs (NSAIDs), vitamin D, selenium, and phytochemicals derived from various fruits, vegetables, and herbs. Investigations are underway to understand their mechanisms of action and evaluate their efficacy in large-scale clinical trials. Additionally, advances in personalized medicine may lead to the identification of genetic markers that can guide targeted chemopreventive strategies.

Chemoprevention, employing drugs and substances to prevent prostate cancer development or progression, offers a promising avenue for prostate cancer prevention. Drugs like finasteride and dutasteride have demonstrated efficacy in reducing prostate cancer risk, while natural compounds like green tea and lycopene show potential in preclinical and epidemiological studies

CHAPTER EIGHT

NUTRITION AND EXERCISE FOR PROSTATE CANCER PREVENTION

Prostate cancer is a prevalent disease, and its incidence continues to rise. While the causes of prostate cancer are complex and multifactorial, lifestyle factors, such as nutrition and exercise, have been shown to play a crucial role in preventing the disease. This article explores the relationship between nutrition and exercise and prostate cancer prevention, highlighting evidence-based dietary recommendations and exercise guidelines. By understanding the current research, men can make informed decisions about their lifestyle choices and take steps towards reducing their risk of prostate cancer.

Research has identified several dietary factors that may contribute to prostate cancer risk. In contrast, others have been shown to reduce the risk of developing the disease. For example, diets high in saturated fats, red meat, and dairy products may increase the risk of prostate cancer, while diets rich in fruits, vegetables, and whole grains may lower the risk.

The Mediterranean diet, characterized by high intake of vegetables, fruits, whole grains, legumes, and olive oil, has been associated with a reduced risk of prostate cancer. Similarly, diets rich in omega-3 fatty acids, found in fatty fish such as salmon, may also offer protection against prostate cancer.

Other dietary components, such as lycopene, a carotenoid found in tomatoes and other red fruits, and green tea, may also have chemopreventive properties against prostate cancer. However, the evidence supporting the role of specific nutrients in prostate cancer prevention is still evolving, and further research is needed to elucidate the optimal dietary patterns for reducing prostate cancer risk.

Physical activity has been associated with a reduced risk of various cancers, including prostate cancer. Regular exercise can help control body weight, reduce inflammation, and improve insulin sensitivity, all of which may contribute to prostate cancer prevention.

According to the American Cancer Society, adults should aim for at least 150 minutes of moderate-intensity or 75 minutes of vigorous-intensity physical activity per week. This can include activities such as brisk walking, cycling, swimming, or strength training. Exercise should be tailored to individual needs and preferences and incorporated into daily routines.

Several studies have shown that exercise can lower the risk of developing prostate cancer and reduce the risk of disease progression in men with prostate cancer. A meta-analysis of 26 studies found that men who engaged in high levels of physical activity had a 10-30% reduced risk of prostate cancer compared to men who were less active.

Combining healthy dietary patterns with regular exercise may offer additional benefits in reducing prostate cancer risk. For example, studies have shown that a plant-based diet combined with regular exercise may have a synergistic effect in reducing the risk of prostate cancer.

Additionally, losing weight through dietary changes and exercise may reduce the risk of developing aggressive prostate cancer. A randomized clinical trial found that overweight and obese men who followed a low-fat diet and engaged in moderate-intensity exercise experienced a 32% reduction in the risk of developing aggressive prostate cancer compared to men in the control group.

Prostate cancer prevention is a complex issue, but lifestyle factors such as nutrition and exercise offer promising avenues for reducing the risk of developing the disease. A healthy diet, including a variety of fruits, vegetables, whole grains, and healthy fats, combined with regular physical activity, can help control body weight, reduce inflammation, and improve overall health. By making informed decisions about their lifestyle choices, men can take steps towards reducing their risk of prostate cancer.

Preferable diet choices and exercises for Prostate Cancer prevention

Mediterranean Diet:

The Mediterranean diet is characterized by high consumption of fruits, vegetables, whole grains, legumes, nuts, and olive oil. It emphasizes lean proteins like fish and poultry over red meat, and moderate consumption of dairy products. This diet is rich in antioxidants, fiber, and healthy fats, which have been associated with a reduced risk of prostate cancer.

Plant-Based Diet:

A plant-based diet focuses on consuming predominantly plant-derived foods such as fruits, vegetables, whole grains, legumes, nuts, and seeds. It limits or excludes animal products, including meat, dairy, and eggs. Plant-based diets are rich in phytochemicals, fiber, and antioxidants, which may contribute to a lower risk of prostate cancer.

DASH (Dietary Approaches to Stop Hypertension) Diet:

The DASH diet is designed to reduce hypertension and improve cardiovascular health. It emphasizes fruits, vegetables, whole grains, lean proteins, and low-fat dairy products while limiting sodium, saturated fats, and added sugars. This diet promotes overall health and may contribute to prostate cancer prevention through its emphasis on nutritious foods.

Low-Fat Diet:

A low-fat diet focuses on reducing the consumption of high-fat foods, including fatty meats, full-fat dairy products, fried foods, and processed snacks. By limiting fat intake, especially saturated fats, this diet may help reduce inflammation and the risk of prostate cancer.

Exercise:

Regular physical activity is crucial for prostate cancer prevention. Engaging in moderate-intensity activities like brisk walking, cycling, swimming, or strength training for at least 150 minutes per week can help control body weight, reduce inflammation, and improve overall health. Exercise also plays a role in managing hormone levels and insulin sensitivity, which are associated with prostate cancer risk.

It is important to note that the effectiveness of specific diets and exercise regimens in preventing prostate cancer may vary among individuals. It is recommended to consult with healthcare professionals or registered dietitians to develop personalized dietary and exercise plans based on individual needs, preferences, and health conditions.

CHAPTER NINE

SUPPORT GROUPS FOR PROSTATE CANCER

Support groups for prostate cancer can be valuable resources for individuals who are diagnosed with the disease, as well as their families and caregivers. These groups provide emotional support, information sharing, and a sense of community with others who are going through similar experiences. Here are some options for finding support groups for prostate cancer:

American Cancer Society (ACS)

The ACS offers a variety of support programs, including in-person support groups for prostate cancer patients. You can visit their website or contact their helpline to find local support groups in your area.

Us TOO International Prostate Cancer Education and Support Network

Us TOO is a nonprofit organization dedicated to supporting men with prostate cancer and their families. They provide in-person and online support groups, educational resources, and advocacy. Their website has a directory of support groups by location.

Prostate Cancer Foundation (PCF)

The PCF provides resources for prostate cancer patients, including online support groups. They have a community section on their website where you can connect with others, share experiences, and ask questions.

Local hospitals and cancer centers

Many hospitals and cancer centers offer support groups specifically for prostate cancer patients. Contact your local medical facilities to inquire about any available support groups or ask your healthcare provider for recommendations.

Online support communities

There are several online platforms where you can find virtual support communities for prostate cancer. Some examples include Cancer Support Community's Cancer Support Helpline, CancerCare's Online Support Groups, and Inspire's Prostate Cancer Support Community.

Remember that support groups vary in terms of their format, frequency, and focus. It's a good idea to explore different options to find a group that meets your specific needs. Additionally, consider reaching out to healthcare professionals, such as oncology social workers or nurses, who may have information on local support resources.

EPILOGUE

Prostate cancer remains a significant health issue, but progress has been made in understanding its effects and advancing prevention strategies. Through early detection, lifestyle modifications, and access to support networks, individuals can navigate the challenges posed by prostate cancer more effectively. Continued research and efforts to raise awareness are vital in improving outcomes and ultimately reducing the impact of this disease on individuals and their communities.